Hormone Fix

Natural Slow Aging Treatment to Balance Your Hormones and Reset Your Metabolism. Proven Healthy Method to Relieve Your Period Pain, Improve Your Sleep Quality and Nurture Your Fertility.

Table of Contents

Introduction: All About Hormones

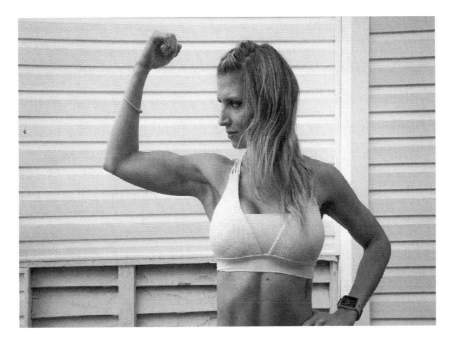

Hormones are chemical substances that all living things produce. They act as the body's "chemical messengers." In most organisms, hormones are produced or formed in one system, but they help various parts of the body to coordinate with each other. The term 'hormone' perfectly suits this chemical substance because it literally means "to set in motion" in Greek.

The existence of hormones was only known in the early 1900s. Since their discovery, scientists have discovered more than 30 hormones in human the human body (Tata, 2005). They have also learned how to extract them in order to start synthesizing them in laboratories. Most of our hormones come from a number of glands in the endocrine system. Some of the main hormone-producing glands include:

- The **adrenal gland** generates the stress hormone and controls sex drive.
- The **hypothalamus** regulates mood, hunger, body temperature, and many more. It's also responsible for stimulating other glands to release hormones.
- The **ovaries** secrete sex hormones, such as estrogen as progesterone.
- The **pineal gland** produces melatonin, the sleep hormone.
- The **pituitary gland** controls all the other glands while producing growth hormones.
- The **testes** produces sperm and testosterone, the male sex hormone.

- The **thyroid gland** produces hormones that are associated with heart rate and calorie burning.

Hormones are responsible for several functions, including reproduction, growth, and development. But for plants, hormones regulate their growth. When your body releases fewer hormones, this may lead to a number of serious conditions and even death.

Some of our organs contain specialized cells that also produce hormones as a response when the regulatory systems of the body send specific signals. For instance, the pancreas generates insulin if the blood sugar level is too high. Depending on how full your intestines are, they also secrete hormones to signal your pancreas or stomach to either increase or decrease their activity. The most important hormones in our body are:

- **Adrenaline** is in charge of the body's fight-or-flight response.
- **Melatonin** is in charge of anticipating darkness each day. This hormone plays a significant role in your energy level throughout the day. It also helps you feel sleepy when nighttime comes.
- **Noradrenaline** controls blood pressure, heart rate, arousal, emotions, etc. Having high levels of this hormone may lead to anxious feelings while low levels of this hormone may lead to depression.
- **Serotonin** controls your mood, sleep cycles, and appetite.
- **Thyroxine** increases your metabolic rate and affects the cells' protein-building process.

The very nature of hormones allows them to become involved in various bodily functions that need coordinated action. They regulate the metabolism and immune system, control growth, and are involved in different developmental phases. Also, hormones influence the timing of cell death. They help us survive through each day by regulating our circadian rhythms with our environment. They provide a much-needed boost to our muscles when our lives depend on it as well. With all these functions etc, it's not really surprising to discover that you can improve or "fix" your life by keeping your hormones healthy.

Since hormones are "signaling" molecules, when you experience hormonal imbalances, these tend to have a negative impact on your organs or systems. For instance, if you suffer from polycystic ovarian syndrome (PCOS), it means that you are also suffering from hormonal imbalance—mainly of the female sex hormones. Because of this, you may experience missed, irregular, or heavy periods, weight gain, excessive hair growth, problems with getting pregnant, acne, etc. When males experience hormonal imbalances, it may cause breast growth, sexual drive reduction, hair loss, muscle and bone mass reduction, and even depression.

These are just some basic examples that demonstrate the importance of our hormones and how important it is for the body to maintain hormonal balance. For most people, their bodies have found ways to maintain this balance naturally. But for others, their hormonal levels are so messed up that they are starting to feel all the negative effects of these imbalances simultaneously. Although we cannot see our hormones, they make life worth living.

This book, *Hormone Fix*, is all about hormones. The different types of hormones, the glands that produce hormones, what happens when you have hormonal imbalances, how to fix those hormonal imbalances—you name it. If you have been feeling not quite right lately, you may blame your hormones. Without even knowing it, you may already be dealing with a number of hormonal imbalances, and you won't start feeling better until you fix them.

Even if you think your hormones are balanced, it's still important to learn all that you can about these chemical substances. That way, in case the symptoms of hormonal imbalances start manifesting themselves, you can recognize them and know exactly what to do to make them right. Learning how to maintain your hormonal balance naturally will also improve your overall well-being. Because of the significance of hormones in the body, educating yourself about them is essential to enrich your life in so many ways!

Chapter 1: How Do Hormones Work?

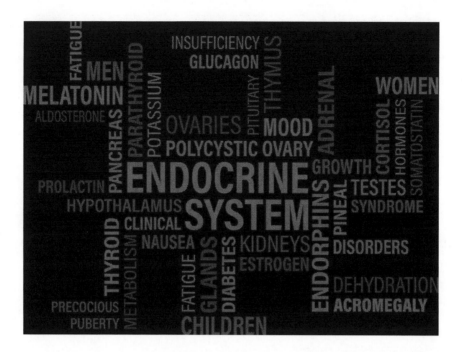

To put it simply, hormones are secreted by the glands and then stored, released, transported, recognized by the cells, relayed, amplified, and broken down. All of these processes allow hormones to do their jobs in order to ensure that your organs are working properly.

For hormones to function, the first thing that happens is secretion. There are different glands that produce these hormones, and the secretion happens as needed. Generally, hormones fall under three main chemical classes: steroids, amino acid derivatives, and eicosanoid hormones. The hormones are first synthesized as pre- or pro-hormones (in an inactive state) by the cells of the glands where they are stored. As soon as these hormones are needed, they are converted into an active state quickly in order to be released.

As soon as the regulatory systems send a signal, indicating a specific requirement that hormones can address, the glands produce the hormones. It can be triggered by different factors like environmental changes, unusual concentrations of specific nutrients or substances, or even other hormones called tropic hormones. The water-soluble hormones enter your bloodstream directly. Once released, they are transported in the blood until they encounter a specific type of receptor protein that's embedded in the cellular membranes or walls. The hormones then bind to these proteins.

The interaction between the hormones and receptor proteins creates an electrical potential which, in turn, triggers a pathway for signal transduction to be activated through the cell membranes. When this happens, "second messengers" are then secreted beyond the membranes to interact with the cells in order to cause the appropriate responses. The system has one significant benefit: it creates cascades of signal transduction to enhance the strength of the first messenger's signal significantly.

On the other hand, far- or lipid-soluble hormones are able to pass through cell membranes so that they can act on the nucleus directly.

As soon as water- or fat-soluble hormones come in contact with proteins, the cells either cease, start, or perform their actions in a different way. Cells can accomplish it through genomic responses, where hormones activate gene transcription to increase the desired protein expression, or non-genomic responses, where actions are performed quickly because they aren't initially or directly influenced by gene expression.

Then, the message gets transmitted, thus causing the cells to start working on their tasks. It allows the regulatory systems to detect the new conditions. They relay these changes back to the glands that can either shut down or adjust the rate of synthesis. After this, the hormones that are already present in the system are broken down to complete the cycle. It's that simple!

Hormone-Producing Glands

Most of the glands that produce hormones are in the endocrine system. It is a glandular network that helps to ensure the proper functioning of the body. The endocrine system is also in charge of regulating a number of internal processes, including:

- Growth
- Development
- Homeostasis
- Reproduction
- Metabolism
- Stimuli responses

The endocrine system is able to accomplish all of these tasks through its glands—the small yet significantly important organs responsible for producing, storing, and secreting hormones. The glands in the endocrine system are:

Adrenal Glands

There are two glands located on top of the kidneys, comprising of two main parts:

1. Adrenal cortex

This is the exterior part of the gland that produces vital hormones like aldosterone, cortisol, etc. It also produces mineralocorticoids and glucocorticoids, such as corticosterone and hydroxycorticosterone. The former is released after the kidney triggers signals while the latter comes after the pituitary gland and hypothalamus trigger signals.

2. Adrenal medulla

Although the functions of the adrenal medulla aren't essential for survival, it does not mean that it's useless. This is the interior part of the gland that produces adrenaline and other non-essential hormones. It releases hormones after receiving stimulation from the sympathetic nervous system, thus helping you deal with emotional and physical stress. The hormones secreted by the adrenal medulla are adrenaline and noradrenaline.

Hypothalamus

This is the part of your brain in charge of maintaining homeostasis—the internal balance of the body. It also happens to be the organ that links your nervous and endocrine systems. It is responsible for inhibiting and releasing hormones that either start or cease the production of other types of hormones throughout your body.

The hypothalamus is involved in the function of your pituitary gland. Upon receiving signals from the nervous system, it secretes neurohormones, substances that either start or cease pituitary hormone secretion. They include:

- Antidiuretic hormone (ADH)
- Corticotropin-releasing hormone (CRH)
- Gonadotropin-releasing hormone (GnRH)
- Growth hormone-releasing hormone (GHRH) or growth hormone-inhibiting hormone (GHIH)
- Oxytocin
- Prolactin-releasing hormone (PRH) or prolactin-inhibiting hormone (PIH)

Ovaries

These maintain reproductive health in females. Apart from producing ova, the ovaries are considered endocrine glands since they also secrete hormones that are crucial to normal fertility and reproductive health.

The main hormones secreted by the ovaries are:

- Estrogen (estradiol, estrone, and estriol)
- Progesterone

Pancreas

This glandular organ maintains the blood sugar level in the body. It functions to release hormones into the bloodstream and enzymes through the ducts. The main hormones secreted by the pancreas are:

- Gastrin
- Glucagon
- Insulin
- Somatostatin
- Vasoactive intestinal peptide (VIP)

Parathyroid Glands

The hormones secreted by these glands regulate the calcium levels in the body. Each parathyroid gland is as small as a grain of rice. Although the glands are located near the thyroid gland, they aren't connected to each other. The only hormone released by the parathyroid glands is the parathyroid hormone (PTH).

Pineal Gland

As tiny as this gland is, it has a very colorful yet misunderstood history. The pineal gland is considered somewhat mysterious as scientists have discovered its functions among all the other endocrine glands. It only secretes one hormone—melatonin—that regulates the body's circadian rhythms as well as specific reproductive hormones.

Pituitary Gland

The pituitary gland is made up of the anterior and posterior lobes, each having its own functions and hormones. The hormones secreted by this "master gland" control how other endocrine glands function. Despite this, it does not really run the show. Here are the main hormones secreted by this gland:

- **Anterior Lobe Hormones:**
    - Adrenocorticotropic hormone (ACTH)
    - Follicle-stimulating hormone (FSH)
    - Growth hormone (GH)
    - Luteinizing hormone (LH)
    - Prolactin
    - Thyroid-stimulating hormone (TSH)

- **Posterior Lobe Hormones:**
    - Antidiuretic hormone (ADH)
    - Oxytocin

Testes

The testes is an organ that produces sperm while maintaining male reproductive health. It secretes one hormone—testosterone—which is important for the normal physical development of young boys. For male adults, this hormone maintains bone density, libido, and muscle strength.

Thymus Gland

The thymus gland is found between the lungs, right behind the sternum. It only remains active until you reach puberty. After this stage of your life, the thymus gland starts to shrink gradually as fat replaces it.

The thymus gland produces a hormone called thymosin. It is responsible for stimulating the development of T-cells that combat diseases. This gland is also important to make sure that the lymphatic system functions well.

Thyroid Gland

The thyroid gland regulates your metabolism. The main hormones it produces are tri-iodothyronine (T3) and thyroxine (T4). When your thyroid gland functions normally, it should produce around 20% T3 and 80% T4 hormones. This gland also generates a hormone called calcitonin that helps regulate the amount of calcium in the body.

Types of Hormones

Hormones are important chemical substances secreted by the glands of the endocrine system that sends messages to different parts of your body. They help manage various processes like sexual desire, blood pressure, hunger, etc. Hormones are flowing throughout your entire body, although they only affect specific cells that can receive their messages.

Throughout the day, you may experience hormonal shifts in your body. As you eat your meals, for instance, your pancreas produces insulin to control your blood sugar levels. When you are at risk of colliding with another car, you tend to slam down on the brakes instantly. At this time, your adrenal glands secrete hormones that allow you to act quickly. At night, your pineal gland gets to work by secreting melatonin so that you can fall asleep easily.

All these things can happen as long as your hormones are balanced. But when you experience an imbalance, you may deal with a number of health issues that may have an adverse effect on your life and health. There are two main types of hormones, namely:

Peptide Hormones

These are protein-based hormones that consist of amino acids. They are dissolvable in water and cannot pass through cell membranes since the latter have a phospholipid bilayer, which prevents the diffusion of fat-insoluble molecules into the cells. Peptide hormones must bind to protein receptors on the surface of cells first to trigger changes within them. This action stimulates the production of a second messenger molecule inside the cell that transports the chemical signal.

Steroid Hormones

These are fat-soluble hormones that can enter the cellular membranes directly. They bind to the receptor cells found in the cytoplasm and carried into the nucleus. Then, the receptors bind to other specific receptors found on the chromatin.

While these are the two main types of hormones, there are many kinds of hormones in the body that are either classified as peptide or steroid hormones. The more you understand them, the easier it will be for you to learn how to balance them.

With that in mind, here are the main hormones in the body:

Adrenaline

This hormone is also known as epinephrine. It is considered as the "emergency hormone" as it initiates quick reactions to be able to think and respond appropriately in emergency situations. When adrenaline is secreted into your body, it increases your metabolism and dilates the blood vessels in your brain and heart. Adrenaline is released into the blood quickly thus, sending impulses to your different organs to create specific responses.

1. Adrenocorticotropic hormone (ACTH)

This hormone stimulates your adrenal glands so that they can start producing hormones that regulate cortisol levels.

2. Androgens

Androgens consist of cholesterol and are found in higher levels in women and other people who experience menstrual cycles. Having excessively high levels of androgen may cause acne, excessive hair growth, infertility, and absent or irregular periods.

3. Antidiuretic hormone (ADH)

This hormone helps increase the kidneys' water absorption into the blood.

4. Corticosterone

This hormone works together with hydrocortisone in the regulation of immune responses and the suppression of inflammatory reactions.

5. Corticotropin-releasing hormone (CRH)

This hormone sends messages to the anterior pituitary gland to stimulate the adrenal glands. This, in turn, causes corticosteroid production to manage immune responses and metabolism.

6. Cortisol

This hormone helps you maintain your health and energy levels as its main role is to control psychological and physical stress. When you experience dangerous or stressful situations, this hormone increases your respiration, blood pressure, and heart rate, among others, as a coping mechanism.

7. Estrogen

Estrogen is mainly associated with menstrual periods, but it also has an effect on vascular, urinary, cardiac, bone, and brain health. Among all the other hormones, estrogen influences people's appearance since it affects body fat composition along with the well-being of the hair and skin.

8. Follicle-stimulating hormone (FSH)

This hormone works with the luteinizing hormone to ensure that the testes and ovaries function normally.

9. Gastrin

Gastrin helps with the digestion process by stimulating specific cells found in the stomach to start producing acid.

10. Glucagon

This hormone works together with insulin to maintain normal levels of glucose by performing contrasting functions of insulin. In other words, it stimulates the cells to release glucose which, in turn, raises your blood sugar levels.

11. Gonadotropin-releasing hormone (GnRH)

The GnRH triggers the production of follicle-stimulating and luteinizing hormones by stimulating the anterior pituitary gland. These two work hand-in-hand to ensure that the testes and ovaries are functioning normally.

12. Growth hormone

This hormone is also called somatotropin. It contains 190 amino acids, which are synthesized and secreted by the cells (somatotrophs) found in the anterior pituitary gland. The growth hormone stimulates cell reproduction and regeneration, growth, and metabolism. Because of these functions, it is crucial for human development.

13. Growth hormone-releasing hormone (GHRH)

This hormone initiates the release of growth hormones by the anterior pituitary gland.

14. Growth hormone-inhibiting hormone (GHIH)

This hormone has the opposite effect as the growth hormone-releasing hormone. In children, the GHIH is essential for the maintenance of their normal body composition. In adults, it affects fat distribution while helping to achieve healthy muscle and bone mass.

15. Hydrocortisone

Hydrocortisone helps regulate how the body converts carbohydrates, proteins, and fats into energy, as well as cardiovascular function and blood pressure levels.

16. Insulin

This hormone enables the body to utilize sugar from carbohydrates. It helps to ensure that your blood sugar levels won't get too high or too low.

17. Luteinizing hormone (LH)

The luteinizing hormone works together with the follicle-stimulating hormone to make sure that the testes and ovaries are functioning normally.

18. Melatonin

This hormone is very special because light dictates its secretion. In the morning, it keeps you alert and awake. But when the night falls and darkness comes, it makes you feel sleepy. It is helpful if you want to control your circadian rhythms and regulate specific reproductive hormones.

19. Noradrenaline

Noradrenaline is also known as norepinephrine, and it works with adrenaline to help the body respond appropriately to stressful situations. However, having too much of this hormone can cause a condition called vasoconstriction in which your blood vessels become narrower, thus resulting in high blood pressure.

20. Oxytocin

This hormone is involved in different bodily processes, such as sleep cycles, orgasms, body temperature, breast milk release, and many more.

21. Parathyroid hormone (PTH)

This hormone has a powerful effect on your bones as it causes the cells there to release calcium into your bloodstream. Parathyroid hormones regulate the amount of calcium that you absorb from the foods you eat, the kidneys excrete, and your bones store.

22. Progesterone

Progesterone promotes pregnancy. The progesterone level remains low during the menstrual cycle up until ovulation. After that, it will rise. This hormone causes changes to the endometrial structure, allowing fertilized eggs to implant. When a woman gets pregnant, this is the main hormone that dominates the body throughout the first trimester. Progesterone also aids in the development of the mammary glands to prepare the body for lactation.

23. Prolactin

This hormone is released after a woman gives birth. The prolactin levels in pregnant women rise during their pregnancy. Ig also plays a significant role in fertility as it may inhibit the gonadotropin-releasing and follicle-stimulating hormones.

24. Serotonin

Serotonin affects the mood; that's why it's considered as a feel-good hormone. Aside from this, serotonin is also associated with memory and learning, sleep and mood regulation, digestion, muscle functions, etc.

25. Somatostatin

This hormone is secreted when the levels of pancreatic hormones such as glucagon and insulin are too high. It helps to maintain the salt or glucose balance in the blood.

26. Testosterone

This is the male sex hormone that helps build muscles and develop the prostate and testes. Testosterone also promotes the development of secondary sexual characteristics like body hair growth, an increase of bone mass, etc.

27. Thymosin

This hormone is responsible for the stimulation of T cell development. All throughout your childhood, lymphocytes (white blood cells) pass through your thymus gland where they get transformed into T cells.

28. Thyroid hormones

These hormones help control the body's metabolism. They also allow you to regular your weight, determine your energy levels and internal body temperature, etc.

29. Thyroid-stimulating hormone (TSH)

This hormone is responsible for the stimulation of the thyroid gland so that it can start producing hormones.

Functions of the Hormones

Hormones are particular types of substances that coordinate the activities of various cells in the body. As mentioned earlier, specific glands in the endocrine system secrete these hormones into the bloodstream. After that, the blood carries hormones to the parts that they are supposed to affect. Generally, hormones have the same significant functions across all living organisms (humans, plants, and animals), such as:

- Assure proper growth from childhood to adulthood
- Ensure adequate maturation and development at the right times
- Ensure that reproduction happens at the best time possible

For all of these functions to occur, the hormones must work together in harmony. This is why hormonal balance is essential. Here are some of the body's major hormones, along with their primary functions:

1. **Adrenaline**
   - Increases blood pressure and constricts the blood vessels (if necessary)
   - Increases heart contractility and heart rate (if necessary)
   - Mobilizes glucose levels
   - Improves blood flow and oxygen utilization
2. **Adrenocorticotropic Hormone (ACTH)**
   - Controls hormone secretion of the adrenal cortex

3. **Aldosterone**
   - Regulates fluid and electrolyte balance
4. **Antidiuretic Hormone**
   - Stimulates kidneys' water retention capability
5. **Cortisol**
   - Increases blood sugar levels
   - Metabolizes CHO, proteins, and fats
   - Inhibits the immune system (if necessary)
   - Has anti-inflammatory effects
6. **Endorphins**
   - Blocks pain
7. **Estrogen**
   - Stimulates the development of sex organs in females
   - Regulates the menstrual cycle
8. **Glucagon**
   - Increases blood sugar levels
   - Stimulates the breakdown of fat and glycogen
9. **Growth Hormone**
   - Stimulates the growth of tissues and organs
   - Increases the synthesis of protein and mobilization and utilization of fat
   - Inhibits the metabolism of carbohydrates
10.   **Insulin**
    - Regulates blood sugar levels (if necessary)
11. **Noradrenaline**
    - Mobilizes glucose
    - Increases heart contractility and heart rate
    - Enhances the utilization of oxygen and blood flow to skeletal muscles
    - Increases blood pressure and narrows blood vessels (if necessary)
12. **Renin**
    - Aids in the regulation of blood pressure
13. **Testosterone**
    - Stimulates the development of sex organs in males
    - Stimulates the growth of facial hair and voice change
14. **Thyroid Stimulating Hormone (TSH)**
    - Regulates thyroid's hormone secretion

Importance of Hormones

Our body consists of a complex network of capillaries, vessels, and other types of structures that communicate and interact with each other and the hormones to ensure that the body functions normally. There are several glands within the endocrine system that release these hormones, and each of them carries out their own tasks.

Hormones are considered as the body's chemical messengers that travel through the bloodstream, your internal "superhighway." While some hormones work quickly to either start or cease certain activities, others constantly work to perform their tasks, such as metabolism, growth and development, reproduction, sexual function, and so on. The hormones are extremely important as they determine your physique, behavior, mood, fertility, digestion, and virtually everything else that goes on in your body.

In order for the body to function optimally, it requires to be in a constant state of hormonal balance. However, if your body experiences any kind of hormonal imbalance, you may experience significant adverse results—unless you fix this imbalance right away. For instance, if you are exposed to extremely cold weather conditions for a long time, your internal temperature will start to fall. To remain healthy, you must maintain a specific body temperature or at least stay within the normal range. This ensures the continuity of your hormonal balance, along with the proper functioning of your organs.

In such a case, your body will work to maintain homeostasis. Certain hormones will be released to specific tissues and cells to stimulate the generation of heat within your body. When this happens, you start experiencing responses such as teeth chattering and shivering. These are essential indications that remind you to wear proper clothes to warm you up or find a warmer location so that your body can start its internal temperature restoration. However, if your internal body temperature continues to drop, and you can't do anything about it, your organs will start failing gradually, too.

This is just one example of what may happen to your body due to environmental changes. Our bodies have different hormones, and some play more critical roles in our well-being than others. If you want to protect your health and manage your condition (if any), understanding your hormones is essential. When your hormones are balanced, they help your body thrive. However, even the smallest imbalances may lead to life-altering and severe symptoms. Therefore, if you have any hormonal issues, it's recommended to consult a qualified endocrinologist.

Chapter 2: Hormonal Imbalances

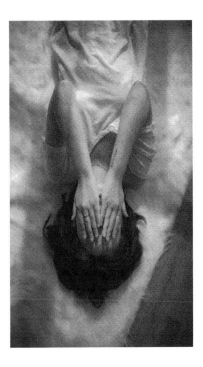

As soon as we are born into the world, our hormones get to work. They influence our sleeping patterns, mood, appetite, stress responses, and everything in between. All these things happen seamlessly unless you experience some internal issues.

You may have already heard the term "hormone imbalance," but do you know what this means?

The term itself sounds so vague and generic that you may not think that it's that big of a deal. But understanding hormone imbalances and what they can do to your body is essential, especially since most of the effects of this condition are detrimental to your health. A hormonal imbalance occurs when there is either too little or too much of a specific hormone in your bloodstream. Since hormones have vital functions, even small problems can cause several side effects throughout your body.

Hormones are vital to regulate some significant processes, such as:

- Appetite
- Metabolism
- Heart rate

- Circadian rhythms
- Sexual function
- Reproductive cycles
- Growth
- Development
- Mood
- Stress levels
- Internal body temperature

With all these etc, you can imagine how much your body will suffer when your hormones are out of whack! Both men and women can experience adrenaline, steroids, growth hormones, and insulin imbalances, among others. Uneven progesterone and estrogen levels are common in women while testosterone imbalances are common in men. While we all experience periods of hormonal imbalances at certain points in our lives, most of us are can bring back that balance without even trying. However, when your endocrine glands aren't functioning correctly or your body cannot deal with the imbalance, that is when you may start experiencing its symptoms, such as:

- Unexplained weight loss or weight gain
- Excessive or unexplained sweating
- Sleeping difficulties
- Changes in your sensitivity to heat and cold
- Changes in your heart rate or blood pressure
- Changes in your body's blood sugar concentration
- Changes in your appetite
- Skin rashes or extremely dry skin
- Puffy face
- Bulge in your neck
- Weak or brittle bones
- Feelings of anxiety or irritability
- Depression
- Long-term and unexplained fatigue
- Frequent headaches
- Increased thirst
- Need to go to the bathroom less or more than usual
- Bloating
- Reduced sex drive
- Infertility
- Brittle and thinning hair
- Blurred vision

- Tenderness of the breast
- Deepening of your voice (for females)

The treatment options when you suffer from a hormonal imbalance would depend on the cause of your condition. Each person may need a different type of treatment for their hormonal imbalance. Some common examples of medications are:

- **Levothyroxine** - improve hypothyroidism symptoms
- **Metformin** - lower or manage blood sugar levels

As mentioned previously, most of us experience at least two periods of hormonal imbalances during our lifetime. These are especially common during pregnancy, menstruation, and puberty. Unfortunately, some people experience irregular or continual hormonal imbalances that throw off their systems, thus causing them to experience several symptoms and side effects.

Often, external factors like hormone medications or stress may cause hormonal imbalances. But there are also cases where medical conditions that involve or affect the endocrine glands or the entire endocrine system make you experience the issue. If you think that you are suffering from some type of hormonal imbalance, therefore, you should speak with your doctor about it. Take note of the symptoms, especially the ones that cause pain or discomfort and interfere with your life.

What Causes Hormonal Imbalances?

The endocrine glands are specialized organs in the body that produce, store, and secrete hormones into the bloodstream whenever necessary. The endocrine system consists of several glands that control various organs. But when these glands secrete too little or too much of these hormones, this is when you experience an imbalance. Most of the time, hormonal imbalances in women are related to their reproductive system. Some of the most common causes are:

- Menopause
- Breastfeeding
- Pregnancy
- Polycystic ovarian syndrome (PCOS)
- Primary ovarian insufficiency
- Premature menopause
- Hormonal medications (such as birth control pills)

Apart from these causes, there are several conditions that may affect the endocrine glands, as well as environmental factors or lifestyle habits that play a role in the development of hormonal imbalances. The chemistry of our bodies is very delicate, after all. Therefore, any factor that alters it can quickly cause noticeable symptoms and health issues. Here are the typical medical conditions, environmental factors, and lifestyle habits that may cause hormonal imbalances:

- High stress levels
- Chronic stress
- Poor sleeping habits
- Unhealthy diet
- Diabetes (types 1 and 2)
- Hyperglycemia
- Hypoglycemia
- Hypothyroidism (underactive thyroid)
- Hyperthyroidism (overactive thyroid)
- Under- or overproduction of the parathyroid hormone
- Poor nutrition
- Being obese or overweight
- Hormone replacement medications
- Abuse of anabolic steroid drugs
- Pituitary tumors
- Solitary thyroid nodules
- Addison's disease
- Cushing's syndrome
- Turner syndrome (in females)
- Prader-Willi syndrome
- Benign cysts or tumors affecting the endocrine glands
- Congenital adrenal hyperplasia
- Endocrine gland injury
- Severe infections or allergic reactions
- Cancers involving endocrine glands
- Radiation therapy
- Chemotherapy
- Iodine deficiency
- Hereditary pancreatitis
- Anorexia
- Exposure to pollutants, toxins, or endocrine-disrupting chemicals like herbicides and pesticides

The foods that you eat may also disrupt your hormonal balance, especially if they cause inflammation. The most common types of foods that can potentially cause this condition are:

- Non-gluten goods
- Dairy products
- Safflower, canola, or sunflower oil

What Happens When You Experience Hormonal Imbalance?

Hormones are no different from the ingredients of a recipe. When you add too much or too little of a certain element, it can affect the overall taste of the dish. While your hormone levels fluctuate throughout your life, especially because of aging, some things cause significant changes and mess up your hormonal balance for an extended period of time. In our cooking analogy, this means that you may have gotten the measurement of an ingredient wrong; that's why it tastes weird.

Our hormones play a vital role in our overall health. When hormonal imbalances occur, you will definitely start feeling its negative effects. We have already gone through the common symptoms experienced by both men and women earlier.

No matter how you look at it, they are very different from each other. From what their likes and dislikes are, how they handle situations, how they express themselves, and many more, these two genders are often as diverse as night and day. As you can probably tell, they are especially different in terms of sex hormones.

Let's look at the hormonal imbalance differences between men and women below.

Hormonal Imbalance in Women

The most common type of hormonal imbalance occurs along with a condition known as polycystic ovarian syndrome (PCOS). Hormonal cycles also tend to fluctuate naturally during puberty, breastfeeding, pregnancy, and menopause. There are several things that may happen to a woman's body that indicate a hormonal imbalance, including

Digestive Issues

Estrogen and other sex hormones affect the microflora in the gastrointestinal tract, as well as the gut function. When these hormones aren't balanced, issues like nausea, diarrhea, constipation, abdominal pain, bloating, and bowel discomfort may appear, especially right before or during the menstrual period.

Excessively Sweaty Skin

Women with hormonal imbalances may also experience excessive sweating because the hormones responsible for controlling the body temperature are not in symmetry.

Extreme Fatigue

Constantly tired women may be suffering from a hormonal imbalance. This may also be caused by high levels of stress and poor sleeping habits.

Hair Loss

While it's normal for us to lose a certain number of hair strands each day, it's not normal for women to start losing chunks of hair. This is one of the more worrying symptoms of hormonal imbalance because no one wants to end up with thinning hair at any age.

An imbalance of thyroid hormones is one of the main causes of hair loss. This may be due to the fact that the thyroid gland isn't functioning properly. Apart from hair loss, a weak thyroid gland may also manifest through dry skin, constipation, and other issues.

Other hormones that may cause hair loss in women include the adrenal and sex hormones.

Loss of Muscle Mass

Not having enough of certain hormones makes it extremely challenging to maintain the strength and muscle mass in women. Fortunately, researchers have discovered that apples and tomatoes may contain compounds that can help prevent or reverse age-related muscle deterioration (Brown, 2015).

Persistent Acne

When women get acne and other skin issues, especially right before they get their periods, it may indicate hormonal imbalance. High testosterone levels in women are associated with acne and similar conditions, after all.

Reduced Sex Drive

The ovaries produce the female sex hormones. Any extreme variations in progesterone and estrogen levels may have a significant effect on a woman's libido.

Unusual and Excessive Weight Gain

When the females' hormones are unbalanced, they typically gain weight or experience difficulty in losing weight. The reason is that high insulin, cortisol, and estrogen levels and low thyroxine levels promote the storage of fats, especially around the abdomen.

Night Sweats and Hot Flashes

These occur in women, especially during the perimenopause stage. Approximately 80% of women in this stage experience night sweats and hot flashes because their hormone levels and cycles are changing (Ferrari, 2015). Women who had their ovaries removed or undergone chemotherapy may experience these symptoms as well because they have low levels of estrogen.

Apart from these effects, other symptoms of hormonal imbalances in women include:

- Missed, stopped, or frequent periods
- Hirsutism (excessive growth of hair on the chin, face, or other in other parts of the body)
- Acne on the upper back or chest
- Skin darkening, especially in the groin, underneath the breasts, and along the neck creases
- Skin tags
- Vaginal atrophy
- Vaginal dryness
- Pain during sex

For women, the main sex hormones are progesterone and estrogen. Estrogen is most associated with women because it plays an important role in puberty and the proper development of girls' reproductive organs. While testosterone is more associated with males, females have them in small amounts, too (while men are dealing with the opposite). Progesterone is also an important sex hormone in women as it prepares their reproductive organs from conception all the way to delivery. Once women reach the age of 40, this hormone starts to wane, which is why most females over that age find it difficult to get pregnant.

Women may experience different types of hormonal imbalances, especially during puberty, menstruation, pregnancy, and menopause. They cause adverse effects on the body, but the good news is that some treatment options are available to help them bring balance back to their hormones. These include:

Anti-androgen medications

They can block the hormone androgen in order to limit excessive hair loss or growth or even severe acne.

Assisted reproductive technology

The most common example of this is in-vitro fertilization (IVF). It may help PCOS sufferers to conceive.

Birth or hormone control

Women who aren't trying to conceive can choose this treatment, which involves taking drugs that contain rogesterone and estrogen to regulate any irregular menstrual cycles and symptoms. Medications can come in the form of shots, patches, pills, rings, or an intrauterine device (IUD).

Clomiphene and letrozole

These drugs can aid with the stimulation of ovulation in women who suffer from PCOS and want to get pregnant. Those with such a condition and other infertility issues may also take gonadotropin injections to increase their chances of conceiving.

Eflornithine

This cream may slow down excessive hair growth in women, especially in the face.

Hormone replacement medication

There are certain medications that may reduce the severe symptoms of menopause—specifically night sweats and hot flashes. However, they are only meant to be taken temporarily.

Vaginal estrogen

This option is for women who experience vaginal dryness due to estrogen level changes. In such cases, women can apply special creams that contain estrogen directly on their vaginal tissues to help reduce the symptoms. They can also use estrogen rings or tablets that offer the same effects.

Hormonal Imbalance in Men

Of course, men experience hormonal imbalances as well. Although it does not happen as frequently as in women, they can manifest through various symptoms. Since testosterone plays a significant role in the development of males, not having enough of this hormone can cause some changes in the body, such as:

- Erectile dysfunction
- Breast tissue development
- Breast tenderness
- Loss of muscle mass
- Reduced sex drive
- Infertility
- Decrease in body hair and beard growth
- Osteoporosis (bone mass loss)
- Hot flashes
- Difficulty concentrating

For men, the three main sex hormones are cortisol, testosterone, and growth hormone. Testosterone is the primary sex hormone in males as it contributes to their bone density, sex drive, muscle mass, and fat distribution. The human growth hormone, on the other hand, is associated with bone and muscle growth, body composition regulation, and proper metabolism. As for cortisol, it helps to control the metabolic rate, blood sugar levels, inflammation, and blood pressure.

Like with women, men also experience hormonal imbalances, especially during puberty and old age because they have different endocrine cycles and organs. There is one very common treatment used for hormonal imbalances: testosterone medications.

We are talking about patches or gels that contain testosterone. These can help reduce the symptoms of conditions that cause low testosterone levels, such as hypogonadism and stunted or delayed puberty.

Hormonal Imbalance in Children and Young Adults

Adult men and women aren't the only ones who can suffer from hormonal imbalances. Even children and young adults may experience this, especially if they are in the pubescent stage. One of the more common conditions caused by hormonal imbalances in children is hypogonadism. Below are its symptoms

- **In young girls**
  - Menstrual period does not start on time.
  - Breast tissues aren't developing
  - There is a delay in growth rate.

- **In young boys**
  - Muscle mass isn't developing well.
  - The voice isn't getting deeper.
  - There is a sparse growth of body hair.
  - The testicular and penis growth is impaired.
  - The limbs (legs and arms) experience excessive growth in relation to the trunk.
  - They experience gynecomastia (breast tissue development).

Common Types of Hormonal Issues

When it comes to hormones, balance is key. There shouldn't be too much or too little hormones in your bloodstream. There should always be the right levels to ensure your overall health and well-being. Generally, when you have yourself checked to determine whether your hormone levels are balanced, this involves basic laboratory tests. If the results of these tests come back and they're not "normal," your doctor may prescribe hormone medications for you. But if your results show that your hormones are balanced, the symptoms you are experiencing may be caused by other issues or medical conditions.

Having an awareness of the different types of hormonal issues can help you catch the symptoms early on. That way, you can consult with your doctor right away to check your hormone levels. Here are some of the most common types of hormonal issues to be aware of:

1. **Cortisol imbalance**

   The adrenal glands are responsible for secreting various hormones, one of which is cortisol—the body's primary stress hormone. When you have an imbalance of this hormone, you may experience a condition known as adrenal fatigue. This occurs when imbalances happen in your cortisol rhythms. Some symptoms of this condition include:

   - Having difficulty "getting started" each morning.

- Always craving for sugary or salty foods.
- A low sex drive.
- Feeling fatigued when afternoon comes but getting a "second wind" when the evening comes.
- You keep waking up at night.
- Feeling dizzy when you stand up quickly.
- Experiencing headaches in the afternoon.
- Issues with your blood sugar levels.
- Chronic inflammation.
- Weakening of the nails.
- Moodiness.
- Finding it difficult to lose weight.

You may experience these symptoms when your cortisol levels are high when they should be low or vice versa. It can also happen that your cortisol levels are always too low or too high. To help overcome this condition, you should mainly focus on minimizing your stress levels.

2. Estrogen imbalance

The balance of the three main forms of estrogen—estrone, estradiol, and estriol—is essential for both men and women. Some symptoms you may experience when you have estrogen imbalances include:

- Hot flashes
- Night sweats
- Vaginal dryness
- Brain fog
- Pain during sex
- Frequent bladder infections
- Constantly feeling lethargic
- Depression
- Feeling bloated and puffy
- Rapid and unexpected weight gain
- Tenderness of the breast
- Mood swings
- Heavy menstrual periods
- Feeling depressed or anxious
- Migraines
- Headaches

- Cervical dysplasia
- Insomnia
- Gallbladder problems
- Constantly feeling emotional and weepy

When imbalances in the levels of these estrogens occur, this may lead to an increase in mortality rates, especially in those suffering from heart disease. It may also hasten the progression of some forms of cancer.

3. Insulin imbalance

Insulin resistance isn't considered a hormonal deficiency. Instead, it's a pattern of hormonal resistance. Insulin resistance is one of the main symptoms of those suffering from type 2 diabetes, but it can also be observed in people who haven't yet progressed to the full-blown disease. Some symptoms you may experience when you have insulin imbalances are:

- Frequently craving sweet foods
- Eating sweet foods do not relieve cravings
- Feeling irritable when you miss meals
- Becoming lightheaded when you miss meals
- Dependence on coffee
- Feeling jittery, shaky or having tremors
- Feeling nervous, agitated or getting upset easily
- Blurred vision
- Poor memory
- Feeling fatigued after meals
- Waist girth is either larger or equal to hip girth
- Frequent urination
- Increased appetite and thirst
- Having difficulties losing weight

One of the main symptoms of prediabetes is resistance to insulin. When this happens, the body produces insulin but it's not utilizing the hormone properly. Unfortunately, the hormone insulin stores fat thus making weight-loss a huge struggle.

4. Leptin imbalance

The fat cells are actually an essential part of your hormonal or endocrine system as they produce leptin, a hormone. If you have leptin imbalance, you may experience symptoms like:

- Being obese or overweight.
- Having difficulties losing weight.
- You crave food constantly.
- You're always stressed out.

One of the main functions of leptin is to tell your brain to utilize the fat stores of the body for energy. But when you suffer from leptin resistance, your body does not recognize this hormone. Therefore, it thinks that it's "starving" so it begins storing your fat.

5. Progesterone imbalance

We all need healthy and balanced levels of progesterone as this hormone helps neutralize the effects and bring balance to the effects of excessive estrogen levels. Some symptoms that may manifest because of an imbalance of this hormone are:

- Insomnia
- PMS
- Painful breasts
- Unhealthy looking skin
- Stubborn and unexplained weight gain
- Anxiety
- Cyclical headaches
- Infertility

Also, without enough progesterone, you may experience estrogen dominance, which is a harmful condition.

6. Testosterone imbalance

In men, low testosterone levels may lead to a greater mortality rate. But over-conversion of testosterone is more common in men. The conversion happens through a process known as aromatization. When the enzyme aromatase experiences excess activities, this causes low levels of testosterone and high levels of estrogen in men. When this happens, it may result in:

- Reduced sex drive
- Erectile dysfunction
- Irritability
- Weight gain
- Enlargement of the breasts

In women, extremely low testosterone levels may cause fatigue, weight gain, a reduction in sex drive, breast cancer, and heart disease. Conversely, when women have high testosterone levels, some symptoms they may experience are:

- Acne
- Excessive growth of hair on the arms and face
- Mid-cycle cramping or pain
- Hypoglycemia
- Infertility
- Thinning hair
- Formation of cysts in the ovaries
- Polycystic ovary syndrome (PCOS)

7. Thyroid imbalance

All of the cells in our bodies require thyroid hormones to ensure their healthy and proper functions. Unfortunately, a lot of underlying thyroid issues aren't detected by standard laboratory tests. Having an imbalance of these hormones may result in the following symptoms:

- Constantly feeling tired
- Feeling cold in your feet, hands or all over your body
- Requiring a lot of sleep in order to function properly
- Weight gain even if you're following a low-calorie diet
- Infrequent and difficult bowel movements
- Depression
- Lack of motivation
- Morning headaches that may wear off as the day progresses
- Thinning of the outer third of the eyebrow
- Thinning of the hair on the scalp
- Excessive hair fall
- Mental sluggishness
- Dry skin

The bottom line is that since the body and all of its hormones are interconnected, having hormonal imbalances may cause effects throughout your body. This is why it's important to maintain hormonal balance at all times. There are many ways to do this—which we will be going through in the next chapters.

Chapter 3: Understanding Your Period

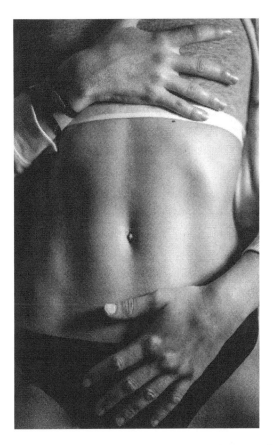

Your period is just one aspect of your menstrual cycle, which refers to the natural changes that a female body goes through in preparation for pregnancy. Usually, the menstrual cycle includes your period—a.k.a. menstruation—which is generally followed by the production of a single egg. During your period, your uterus discharges cells, mucus, and blood. The menstrual cycle begins on the first day and ends before your next period starts. The typical length of a cycle is 28 days, but it varies between women. When your menstrual cycle lasts between 20 to 40 days, this is still normal. However, when it exceeds more than six weeks, this is already considered unusual.

In adolescent women and those approaching menopause, meanwhile, experiencing irregular periods is common. Other factors that may cause irregular periods are extreme emotions (whether bad or good), high stress levels, traveling, and excessive physical activities.

To understand your menstrual cycle better, you should know precisely what happens during its stages.

Follicular Phase

The pituitary gland releases follicle-stimulating hormone during the follicular phase. When this happens, it causes follicles—cells containing immature eggs—to start developing in the ovaries. These also produce oestrogen, which causes a thickening of the uterus. It helps to prepare for the possibility of a fertilized egg getting embedded in that part.

In most women, only one follicle can reach full maturity. It then moves to the surface of the ovary while the other follicles are broken down and reabsorbed by the body. This phase starts on the first day of a period and ends when the ovulation phase begins.

Ovulation Phase

Ovulation occurs when a mature egg leaves the ovary. Before this, the oestrogen levels of women increases and causes the brain to release the gonadotropin-releasing hormone. The latter stimulates the pituitary gland to start producing higher levels of luteinizing hormone that triggers ovulation. After ovulation, the egg gets swept into the fallopian tube before moving towards the uterus. If the egg isn't fertilized, it disintegrates within 6 to 24 hours.

Just before this phase occurs, the cervical mucus becomes slippery and clear, like the white part of a raw egg. It becomes very elastic, and you can even stretch it into a string between your fingers. This is known as "fertile mucus" since women are considered fertile when it is present. This type of mucus nourishes and aids the sperm that travels towards the cervix's opening.

During the non-fertile phase of a woman's cycle, the cervical mucus has a different texture and color. It may be gummy, creamy, sticky, or crumbly. Its color may be yellow, white, or milky. Unlike the fertile mucus, you cannot stretch this between your fingers, and its smell is somewhat sour. The appearance of your cervical mucus can be affected by lubricants, semen, sexual arousal, vaginal infections, and some types of medications.

Both the opening and positioning of the cervix may change throughout your cycle. During the ovulation phase, it is in a higher position and has a broader entrance. In some cases, women experience pain or aches during this phase of their menstrual cycle. The ovulation period typically begins 12 to 16 days before the start of the next period. Women who have regular menstruation cycles may find it easier to approximate their ovulation time. This becomes significant for women who are trying to get pregnant. After ovulation, the lifespan of the mature egg is between 6 to 12 hours, but for some women, this can last up to 24 hours.

Luteal Phase

During the luteal phase, any remaining follicles—a.k.a. corpus luteum—start releasing large amounts of progesterone along with oestrogen. This process contributes to the uterine lining's further maintenance and thickening. Without fertilization, the corpus luteum break down and causes a decline of progesterone levels and thinning of the uterus lining. During this phase, you may experience physical and emotional changes, as well as fluid retention, tiredness, lumpy or tender breasts, mood swings, bloating, and even anxiety.

Menstruation

The menstruation stage occurs as the lining of the uterus, which has been broken down, flows out of the vagina. Usually, a woman's period lasts between 3 to 7 days, but the duration may vary from one woman to another and from one cycle to another. Aside from blood, the menstrual fluid that comes out of the vagina includes cervical mucus, vaginal secretions, and endometrial cells.

Most women lose around 50 to 100 mL of fluid during menstruation. The amount of menstrual flow may vary throughout a woman's cycle, while the color of the fluid may range between bright red, dark red, pink, black, and brown.

What Your Period Should Be Like

Once every month, women who have already undergone puberty will get their periods. It occurs as the uterine lining has more blood vessels and gotten thicker in preparation for the possibility of getting pregnant. If the egg remains unfertilized after a few hours, the broken down uterus lining will shed along with other fluids through the vagina. For most women, periods occur in a relatively predictable and regular pattern.

The entire cycle is regulated by a complex group of hormones that are produced by the hypothalamus, pituitary gland, and ovaries. Periods are a healthy and regular part of the menstrual cycle, and the first day of your period also signifies the start of a new menstrual cycle. All women should observe their menstruation as it can be a significant indicator of your health. You should know precisely what a "normal" period is like and what a "normal" period is for you. In this case, it refers to the frequency of your periods, how heavy or light your periods are, and how long your periods last.

When it comes to bleeding during menstruation, there is a normal range. While some women experience long, heavy periods, others have shorter and lighter ones. Over time, you may also notice changes, here are a couple of things that a lot of women deal with:

- Each period comes every 21 to 35 days. You can count from the first day of your current period to the first day of your next period.

- Although the total amount of blood excreted during the period may only be around 2 to 3 tablespoons, the secretion of other fluids makes it seem like you are producing a lot more.

You may experience fluctuations in your periods after menarche (your first period), after giving birth, or as you approach menopause. During these times, anovulation—irregular ovulation—is quite common and can even cause heavy or absent periods temporarily. If you do not undergo the ovulation phase during each menstrual period, you may miss your period or it may come late, shorter or longer, or lighter or heavier than your regular periods.

Between these stages of your life, your period should be approximately the same volume and length for each menstrual cycle. However, you may experience changes when you are dealing with specific types of hormonal imbalances. Remember, your hormonal levels may temporarily change because of many factors, such as your diet, stress, exercise, etc. Just as each woman's body is different, each period is different as well.

Of course, these "normal" periods do not apply to the ladies who are taking birth control. Nowadays, there are so many types of hormonal birth control, all of which contain varying levels and types of hormones. Let's take a look at some of the most common birth control options and how they affect your menstrual periods:

Copper IUD

This is non-hormonal; thus, you may experience the same progesterone and estrogen fluctuations throughout your menstrual cycle. However, most women who use a copper IUD experience more extended period length and a heavier menstrual flow, especially within the first 6 to 12 months of using the device. This happens because of vascular changes, as well as changes in uterine blood flow. Also, cramping and large clots may accompany menstrual bleeding.

Hormonal IUD

When using this device, it's common for women to experience either light or irregular bleeding. For some , their bleeding stops entirely because the uterine lining does not thicken enough. This is especially true for those who use hormonal IUD for several months or years.

Mini Pill

When you use progestin-only pills for birth control, you may not experience regular menstrual cycles. Some of them tend to suppress the process of ovulation. When it comes to progestin-only contraceptives, bleeding may vary as well. Any changes that happen in your period occur in response to your body's hormonal changes. These hormones affect your uterine lining growth and shedding. Irregularities in your period are especially common when you do not take the pills at the same time each day.

Shot and Implant

These methods also tend to suppress the process of ovulation. Because of these birth control methods, you may not ovulate regularly. Because of this, you may experience lighter, shorter, or occasionally absent periods, but it does not happen for all women. Also, irregular spotting and prolonged bleeding are relatively common, especially at the beginning. Over time, the symptoms may improve in some women but continue in others.

Apart from your periods, it's also essential for you to look out for any bleeding that occurs when you are not menstruating. This is called "spotting" and is caused by different reasons, such as ovulation bleeding, hormonal birth control, and other physiological issues. If you notice that you are experiencing spotting frequently, consult your healthcare provider right away to determine the cause of your spotting and how to deal with it.

The Role of Hormones in Your Period

Hormones play an important role in your whole menstrual cycle. We have already discussed the different phases of the latter. Now, let's go through them again, but this time, let's focus more on the hormones involved in each phase, as well as how you may feel during these phases.

Follicular phase

During this phase, you would feel like you're at your best. You have low progesterone levels and high estrogen levels, thus giving you elastic and glowing skin along with an overall energized and fresh feeling.

Early in the follicular stage, high FSH levels trigger a process called folliculogenesis. In the beginning, several follicles grow simultaneously, but only one dominant follicle is chosen. Follicles that grow into maturity start producing estrogen, which elevates the levels of luteinizing hormones. When the latter and estrogen levels are high, they trigger complex biochemical reactions, thus leading to ovulation.

During the follicular phase, you will feel very positive between the 6th and 14th days of your menstrual cycle. You may feel more confident as your testosterone and estrogen levels peak. Knowing this can give you an edge, especially when you time interviews, presentations, and other activities that require confidence around this time. Also, during this time, your skin may give off a natural scent induced by your hormones; therefore, you may want to go easy when using cologne or perfume.

Ovulation Phase

This is the phase when the chosen dominant follicle releases an egg that can potentially be fertilized by sperm. If you want to get pregnant, the most significant change would be on the 14th day before the start of your next menstrual cycle. As soon as your levels of estrogen peak, your luteinizing levels also rise because of positive feedback. This occurrence triggers ovulation, along with the release of an egg from your ovary.

The main change you may notice during this phase is in your vaginal secretion. Your cervical mucus turns into fertile mucus, which is clearer, more elastic, and with an increase in the quantity. However, if you start feeling particularly sensitive or sore or you notice excessive amounts of vaginal secretion, you may want to get yourself checked as you may have some underlying issues.

Luteal Phase

During the luteal phase, your estrogen and luteinizing hormone levels start going down. The dominant follicle gets transformed into a corpus luteum before breaking down. For most women, the luteal phase lasts for about 14 days as your body prepares itself for possible implantation. Your progesterone levels may start going up, and this is the time when you may start experiencing PMS symptoms.

Most women do not feel too good during this phase since it may cause skin issues, irritability, and negative moods. Sometimes, high levels of progesterone may also cause constipation. Other common symptoms you may feel during the luteal phase include:

- An increase in your appetite
- Breakouts
- Tiredness or fatigue
- Oily skin and hair

While some women won't feel any physical changes because of their fluctuating hormone levels, others experience severe symptoms that may interfere with their lives. For that reason, learning how to deal with the symptoms can make your life easier etc comfortable even as you go through the different phases of your menstrual cycle.

Menstruation

Unless fertilization occurs, you may experience more shifts in your hormone levels late in the luteal phase. Specifically, your hormone levels may start going down while your prostaglandin levels may start going up. Because of these changes, the contraction of the uterine muscles occurs while the inner uterine layer sloughs. This is when menstrual bleeding or menstruation occurs.

The hormone levels that start going down are those of estrogen and progesterone. When this happens, you may experience other menstrual symptoms like breast and skin tenderness, tiredness, migraines, cramping, headaches, mood swings, and lower back pain. Also, during menstruation, you may feel uncomfortable and have a bad mood overall. The good news is that there are certain things that you can do or foods that you can eat to make you feel better.

In some cases, women may suffer from intensely painful cramps during menstruation. For this, you may take OTC painkillers or apply a heating pad on your abdomen or lower back to ease the pain.

What Is Premenstrual Syndrome?

Most women experience specific symptoms that indicate the incoming period. For most women, simple symptoms like mild breast tenderness or craving for sweet foods aren't that big of a deal. But for others, severe symptoms interfere with their routine. If you experience such symptoms, you may have a premenstrual syndrome or PMS. This is a condition wherein you experience behavioral, emotional, or physical symptoms around 1 to 2 weeks before you get your period. Once your menstrual period starts, though, these symptoms stop as well.

The PMS symptoms appear around the 14th day of your menstruation cycle and last until a week after your period begins. Again, the severity of the symptoms may vary depending on the month or individual. The most common ones are:

- Abdominal bloating or pain
- Breast soreness
- Acne
- Food cravings, especially sweet foods
- Constipation or diarrhea
- Headaches
- Irritability
- Sensitivity to sounds or lights
- Fatigue
- Changes in sleep patterns
- Sadness
- Depression
- Anxiety

- Emotional outbursts

Although PMS is a common condition in women, doctors do not really know its exact cause. However, people believe that the changes in body chemistry and hormonal levels that occur around the time of your menstrual period triggers the symptoms. There are also some risk factors that may trigger or worsen your PMS, including:

- Smoking
- Stress
- Lack of exercise or physical activity
- Lack of sleep
- Overconsumption of alcohol
- Eating too much red meat, sugar or salt
- Depression

If your PMS causes mood swings, physical pain, and other debilitating symptoms—or if the symptoms do not go away even after your period starts—consult a doctor. You can receive a proper diagnosis if you are experiencing more than one of these symptoms. Also, your physician may be able to rule out other conditions that may have the same symptoms, such as:

- Endometriosis
- Anemia
- Thyroid disease
- Chronic fatigue syndrome
- Irritable bowel syndrome (IBS)
- Rheumatologic or connective tissue diseases

To come up with a proper diagnosis, your doctor may ask you some questions about your medical or family history to determine whether PMS is causing the symptoms or there is a possibility that you're suffering from another health issue. Some of the tests are pelvic exam, pregnancy test, and thyroid hormone test.

Tips and Strategies for Restoring Your Regular Periods

There are many reasons why you experience period irregularities. Having irregular or missing periods is a common thing in women of all ages. When your period stops completely, this means that you are either pregnant, breastfeeding, or menopausal. In some cases, engaging in frequent and intense exercise routines can interfere with your menstrual cycle as well. If you are underweight or overweight or have PCOS, you may not be able to enjoy regular menstrual periods either. Of course, when you use hormonal birth control, irregular menstruations may be one of the side effects. Even after you stop using birth control, it won't guarantee that your period will come back right away.

While there are common and known causes of irregular or missing periods, some lesser-known causes of this condition exist as well. One of them is chronic stress. When you are always stressed, you tend to have high levels of cortisol in your body. This, in turn, throws your blood sugar off balance, thus disrupting your ovulation. Some studies have shown that women who work in stressful environments or have stressful jobs are at an increased risk for anovulation and irregular menstrual periods (Allsworth et al., 2007). This may also make it difficult for such women to get pregnant.

Another overlooked cause of irregular and missing periods is blood sugar dysregulation. This condition may lead to infertility. In some cases, doctors may prescribe specific diabetes medications to women who have blood sugar dysregulation to stimulate ovulation. While these medications may work, there are safer, natural remedies that may help you restore your regular periods:

Try doing yoga

Several studies have shown that yoga is an effective natural treatment for different types of menstrual problems (Rani et al., 2011). Doing 30 to 40 minutes of yoga around five times each week for several months can help bring balance to hormonal levels that are related to missing or irregular periods. Besides, yoga can also reduce emotional symptoms and menstrual pain that are often associated with menstrual periods. Doing yoga may improve your quality of life, especially if you suffer from dysmenorrhea.

The great thing about yoga is that there are poses and routines for people of different levels. As a beginner, you can start with the simple ones and then move on to more complex ones as you progress. You can also do yoga at home or in studios depending on your comfort level, free time, and lifestyle.

Make self-care your priority

If you want to enjoy regular periods, then it's time to focus on self-care. Make relaxation one of your goals since stress is one of the significant (yet relatively unknown) causes of irregular or missed periods. While yoga can help you relax, there are other things you can do to make your life less stressful. Treat yourself to massages and different types of spa treatments once in a while. Engage in leisure activities that you enjoy. Take time off for yourself and do things that make you feel relaxed. And most of all, do not feel guilty about prioritizing self-care.

Taking care of yourself helps balance your hormones and improves your overall well-being.

Achieve and maintain a healthy weight

Weight is another factor that may affect the regularity of your periods. If you are obese or overweight, shedding those excess pounds may help regulate your menstrual periods. Conversely, being underweight or losing too much weight can also cause irregularities in your menstrual periods. This is why you need to know your ideal weight, work hard to achieve it, and maintain that weight.

Stabilize blood sugar levels

One of the most effective ways to deal with blood sugar issues is to follow a healthier diet. Opt for healthy carbohydrate food sources, along with healthy proteins and fats. Also, load up on non-starchy veggies in different colors at each meal. When you're able to stabilize your blood sugar levels, this may help give you regular periods too.

Exercise regularly

Most health problems can be improved through regular exercise. It does not mean that you should start a high-intensity exercise routine that you force yourself to do each day, though. Doing this may worsen your condition and cause your periods to stop altogether! Instead, you should try to tailor your exercise routines to your own needs and capabilities. do not push yourself too hard, especially if you haven't been exercising in the past. Start with light exercises to get your heart pumping. Over time, you can increase your workout routines until you find that "sweet spot" that makes you feel happy and healthy and makes your periods more regular.

Get enough sleep each night

When you do not get enough sleep each night, this causes detrimental effects to your hormonal balance, period, and health. We all have natural circadian rhythms that allow us to stay alert and energized in the morning and sleep restfully at night. But when you are short on sleep, or you always have poor sleeping habits, it becomes virtually impossible to bring and maintain hormonal balance.

To fix this issue, make sure that you are getting enough sleep each night. If you think it will help, come up with your bedtime routine to tell your body and brain that it's time to wind down and prepare to rest. This may take some getting used to, but if you can improve your sleeping habits, you will notice some improvements in your health and period.

Chapter 4: Hormones and Aging

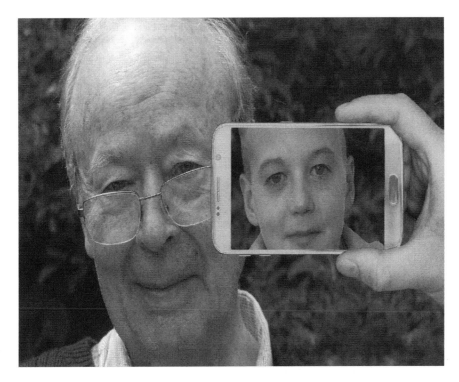

One common misconception about hormones that a lot of people believe is that they only affect our emotions. A lot of perceptions and myths are about teenagers who are regularly experiencing problems with their attitudes and behaviors, which they blame on hormones. Sometimes, people also believe that women go through emotional outbursts right around a particular time of the month because of hormones. While it's true that the latter can affect these responses, there is so much more to them than that.

Our hormones affect growth, development, functions of different body parts, and even the process of aging. When it comes to longevity and trying to delay the aging process, maintaining the proper balance of hormones throughout your body is critical. When your hormone levels are balanced, your body can produce essential nutrients and functions needed for long-term mental and physical well-being. In other words, hormones can control the aging rate. When there is a decrease in the hormone production of certain glands, this may cause depression, bone and muscle loss, and slow bodily processes.

While most hormone levels naturally decrease with age, certain hormones remain at stable levels while others may even rise. But even if your hormone levels do not go down, the functions of your endocrine system may decline as you grow older. It happens when hormone receptors lose their sensitivity. Some of the primary hormones that decrease with age are:

- Melatonin
- Growth hormone
- Estrogen (in females)
- Testosterone (in males)

A decrease in the levels of melatonin may affect your circadian rhythms. When growth hormone levels go down, this leads to a reduction in your muscle strength and mass. For women, when their estrogen levels decline, this results in menopause. But for men, the decrease in their levels of testosterone happens slowly.

The main hormones that only decrease slightly or remain unchanged are:

- Thyroid hormones
- Insulin
- Cortisol

Then, some hormones may increase as you grow older, such as:

- Luteinizing hormone
- Follicle-stimulating hormone
- Parathyroid hormone
- Adrenaline
- Noradrenaline

While hormone replacement therapy may benefit you later, especially when you start experiencing a decrease in functions, It does not seem to prolong life or reverse the aging process. It can even cause harm in some cases, such as when older women opt for estrogen replacement. Although a reduction in hormone production is inevitable, there are ways to restore it and bring back your hormonal balance. This is especially beneficial in terms of preventing the development of several medical conditions. But before we go into these practical and helpful tips, let's learn about how your hormones affect the aging process and vice versa.

What Happens to Your Hormones When You Age?

Hormones are utilized by target systems and organs in the body. Hormones control them so that they can perform their functions well. Some even possess their own control systems that work either in place of or alongside the hormones. In most cases, target tissues lose some of their sensitivity to the hormones that regulate them. There may also be changes in the number of hormones that the glands produce.

As you grow older, some blood levels of hormones may increase, decrease, or remain the same. Their metabolism may slow down as well. Since many organs that are responsible for producing hormones are controlled by hormones, a ripple effect happens as you age. Let's take a look at the most significant hormonal changes that occur when you are older:

Hormonal changes

Both men and women will experience hormonal changes as they age--this is a fact of life. This may happen for a number of reasons apart from the natural age-related decline of the body and its systems. Some changes you may notice are:

- By the time you reach middle age, your pituitary gland would have already peaked in terms of size. From there, it starts growing smaller.
- Our endocrine organs may respond differently to the hormones that control them. Therefore, even if your hypothalamus produces the same amount of regulating hormones, you may still experience imbalances.
- As you age, your levels of parathyroid hormones may increase, which contributes to the development of osteoporosis.
- The thyroid gland produces hormones that regulate muscle strength, body temperature, metabolism, and many more. Therefore, when you suffer from a disease that affects this gland, you may experience a lot of physical changes.
- Once you reach the age of 50, you will start experiencing an increase in your levels of fasting glucose. It happens because your cells lose their sensitivity to insulin.
- The adrenal glands may not be able to produce enough of the hormone aldosterone, which helps regulate the balance of electrolytes and fluids. Because of that, you may deal with lightheadedness or a condition known as orthostatic hypotension (a sudden drop in your blood pressure) when you change position suddenly.

These are some of the most noticeable changes that come with age. In order to prevent them from happening, a healthy lifestyle is key. This may help slow down the natural decline of your body, along with the numerous effects that it may have on your hormones and the glands that generate them.

Andropause

This is a condition that most but not all men experience. It occurs when there is a dramatic decrease in the body's testosterone production. While the common belief is that andropause is the "male menopause," it really isn't. Some of the more common symptoms of this condition are:

- Cognitive impairment
- Increased risk of developing osteoporosis
- Bone mineral density reduction
- Erectile dysfunction
- Decreased libido
- Depression
- Muscle mass reduction
- Reduced energy
- Decrease in overall strength

When it comes to this condition, a mere 20% of 60-year-old males and over would experience it. For older males who to beyond the age of 80, it is more common as it occurs more frequently.

Menopause

When women reach the age of 50, the ovaries start to reduce their progesterone and estrogen production. When it happens, the pituitary gland compensates for these hormonal reductions by providing more follicle-stimulating hormones. For this condition, women may experience varying symptoms, such as:

- Vaginal atrophy
- Vaginal dryness
- Painful intercourse
- Hot flashes
- Insomnia
- Reduced libido
- Depression
- Irritability
- Osteoporosis

While some medications may help ease these symptoms, research has shown that taking them may cause a higher risk of blood clots, breast cancer, cardiovascular disease, and stroke (Humphries & Gill, 2003). To be safe, you may take such medications (after consulting with your doctor) for a short period only--just enough to help with the transition.

What Happens to Your Hormones in Your 20s?

When your hormones are balanced, it's like they are all part of a professional orchestra playing beautiful music. But when you lose this balance, your orchestra becomes a discordant symphony. Following this analogy, when your hormones play too soft or loud, too slow or fast, and do not cooperate with other hormones, they may have jarring effects on your body. Fortunately, while you are still young—like when you are in your 20s—your hormones are still at their peak.

While you may enjoy hormonal balance in your 20s, the modern world makes it quite difficult to maintain it due to various environmental factors, e.g., harmful chemical and toxin exposure, extreme stress, unhealthy food options, and many more. Despite that, you should be aware of the health of your hormones as early as when you reach this age. After all, this sets the stage for your overall—and future—wellness. In particular, women should place a lot of importance in their hormones during their 20s because they undergo important phases in their lives.

During the menstrual years, women may experience plenty of stressors—both good and bad. In your 20s, you may move to a new place, go to graduate school, find your first job, have your first taste of alcohol or caffeine, etc. Whether you experience stressful or exciting changes in life, these will affect your hormonal balance significantly. This may also be a time when you observe new issues with your period or a continuation of symptoms you have had during puberty.

In order to address any hormonal imbalances in your 20s, you need to pay attention to your toxin exposure and diet. If you want your hormones to remain healthy and balanced as you progress to the next phase of your life, make sure that you are getting all the essential micronutrients that your body needs to thrive. Also, you should try to sync your exercise routines with your menstrual cycle.

When women get pregnant, their hormone sensitivity indicates the degree to which they can deal with hormonal symptoms during their menstrual years. It is possible to feel amazing during pregnancy, you just need to prepare for it by making lifestyle and diet changes months before they even try to conceive. This is even more important for hormonally sensitive people since hormone levels tend to surge during pregnancy, which may lead to a number of health issues.

The diet that you have been following for the past decade before getting pregnant may put you at risk for developing postpartum depression. If you want to prevent this from happening, you should—again—take care of yourself early. This is why self-care is crucial for both men and women. Postpartum depression is a real thing, and it is extremely difficult to deal with. Nevertheless, caring for your hormones can help reduce your hormone sensitivity so that you can lower your risk of developing this condition.

What Happens to Your Hormones in Your 30s?

When you reach your 30s, this time may feel somewhat bittersweet. As you are finding your own identity, your body may start showing the initial yet subtle signs of the aging process. As you gradually achieve stability in your personal and professional life, you may discover that this newfound stability may also come with its own set of stresses and challenges. Apart from these, you may also feel stressed by the hormonal changes that take place in your body.

If you expose yourself to too much sun or you have had a little too much fun during your adolescence or young adulthood, your 30s is the time when you have to pay the price. If you have lived a healthy and happy life, expect to notice wrinkles forming in the areas around your eyes. These are the "wrinkles of joy" that have formed naturally as you age since your skin becomes less regenerative and less elastic with the passage of time. You may also see the common signs of aging earlier if you spent a lot of hours out in the sun without using skin protection such as sunscreen.

For women, one typical stressor is being able to stay fit, especially for those who have already given birth in their 20s or early 30s. Moms may find it difficult to manage parenting, career, relationships (with their partner, family, and friends), home, and so on. With all of these things going on in their lives, it can be extremely challenging to maintain a lean, strong, and fit body. When you are in your 30s, therefore, it becomes even more essential to exercise regularly in order to keep your hormones balanced, regardless of your gender.

Again, for women, 30s is a crucial time for hormones, especially if you want to get pregnant at this age. As they progress through this phase, they continue with the reproductive continuum path. While it is easier for most women to conceive during their 20s, they may have already shed approximately half of their viable eggs. This is why it is more difficult for those aged 30+ to get pregnant. The process of trying can be both emotionally and physically challenging; the risk of pregnancy complications, miscarriage, and birth defects increases as well.

Hormonal changes during this phase may cause significant changes to a woman's menstrual cycle, too. They may experience heavier periods due to uterine tumors known as fibroids that aren't cancerous. For women who have already given birth, they may deal with some level of

46

urinary incontinence as well. Others experience perimenopause when they reach the age of 35 and above. This is another condition that causes a lot of hormonal changes and physical symptoms.

For both men and women, the hormones responsible for building muscles (e.g., testosterone and growth hormone) start going down. It causes muscle loss and a slower rate of metabolism, which may result in weight gain.

What Happens to Your Hormones in Your 40s?

Turning 40 does not mean that you have to experience a midlife crisis. While many people go through emotional and physical changes around this age, there are different ways to mark this milestone as the start of your best years and embrace the new journey ahead.

As soon as you reach the age of 40, you may start noticing even more changes in your life and body. You may be feeling "in-between"--meaning, not young anymore but not quite old yet. Deep inside, your hormone levels are starting to fluctuate more frequently. Despite your healthy diet and regular exercise efforts, you may notice that you are gaining weight as well. There may be times when you feel annoyed, tired, or short, and you may see that your sleeping patterns have changed.

For women, when they reach 40, they feel too young to experience the symptoms of menopause. However, a lot of them deal with pre-menopausal or perimenopause signs since the latter generally manifest about 8 years before menopause. While bothersome, the symptoms are often perceived as a "normal part" of the process. Perimenopause can take place when the levels of FSH start rising to the point that ovulation does not occur anymore. However, for some women who have experience hormonal imbalances during the first stage of menopause, they may experience unnecessarily complicated symptoms and health issues.

When you have balanced hormones in your 40s, your body will still be able to produce testosterone, estrogen, and progesterone, albeit in lesser amounts. If you experience the common symptoms of perimenopause or menopause (e.g., night sweats, hot flashes, no libido, etc.), you may want to try making adjustments to your lifestyle and diet until you have eased the symptoms and feel better.

One of the worst parts of hormonal imbalance is the disruptions in your sleeping patterns. When you cannot sleep well each night, it won't just leave you feeling fatigued. It may also lead to weight gain as the production of ghrelin (the hunger hormone) increases while the creation of leptin (the appetite-suppressing hormone) decreases. Hormones can also contribute to the development or worsening of sleep apnea, another sleep-related problem.

As you grow old, it becomes even more essential to take care of yourself, so make sure that you are getting your hormone levels checked regularly. Also, invest in self-care as things may get even more difficult beyond this phase of your life. Of course, this does not have to be the case if you try your best to keep your hormones balanced.

Can Healthy Hormones Slow Down the Aging Process?

Have you ever heard the saying, "With age comes wisdom?" Wisdom is excellent, and we would all love to have more of it. However, other things come with age, such as ailing joints, general frailty, wrinkles, and many more. As simple as it may seem, the key to aging well is right in front of you—or at least, within you. Your hormones!

While the hormones that are commonly associated with aging are DHEA and the growth hormone, others play an essential role in the process, too. If any of these hormones go out of whack, it can affect your body negatively and even make you age faster than ever. Here are the hormones that cause the latter, as well as tips on how you can keep them balanced and healthy to avoid aging faster:

Cortisol

Stress affects the skin cells by inducing significant collagen loss, which reduces the elasticity of the skin. Since cortisol is the stress hormone, having high levels of it may speed up the aging process. Therefore, you must learn how to manage your stress more effectively.

DHEA

This is a precursor hormone that is produced by the adrenal glands from cholesterol. DHEA plays a vital role in testosterone and estrogen production. It also stimulates the physical transformations that you go through as you mature. By your mid-20s, your DHEA levels may start to decline gradually, thus contributing to the aging process. By the time you reach 70 years old, you may have less than 10% of this hormone than when you were in your 20s.

Undergoing therapy that involves DHEA may be beneficial to treat several medical conditions that come with age. This may also help you balance your DHEA levels to improve your overall health.

Estrogen

For most women, their estrogen levels may begin to decline in their mid-40s. But for those who are very thin, lead a stressful lifestyle, sick, have irregular eating habits, and hardly get enough sleep, their estrogen levels may go down much sooner. When this happens, it makes the skin less elastic and thinner, thus resulting in sagging and wrinkling. You can improve your estrogen levels by taking estrogen supplements or learning how to take care of your hormones.

Growth Hormone

The growth hormone is essential for the development and maintenance of your tissues and organs. It enhances the growth of your tissues, increases your muscle mass, and even makes your bones stronger. With all of these functions, having imbalanced levels of growth hormones will lead to poor health and faster aging process.

Insulin

The higher your insulin levels are, the faster wrinkles may appear on your skin. Your body may start producing excessive amounts of insulin when you always indulge in high-carb and high-sugar foods.

If you want to avoid this, you may want to follow a healthier, balanced diet in which you focus on healthy fats, lean proteins, and minimal carbs. It is also a good idea to wait for at least 3 to 4 hours between meals to maintain your insulin levels.

Melatonin

Melatonin is a type of antioxidant hormone that protects your body against UV radiation. It also plays a role in repairing skin damage and slow down the aging process.

Without adequate sleep or protein in your system, your melatonin levels may drop. To replenish your melatonin levels, you should consume enough protein and opt to take supplements either orally or topically.

Progesterone

For both men and women, this hormone serves several functions in the body. To be precise, it regulates sleep cycles, boosts brain function, enhances immunity, and many more.

Progesterone is essential for the reproductive processes in women, too. Any imbalance concerning this hormone may result in mood swings, foggy thinking, poor sleep, and the emergence of the common signs of aging.

Testosterone

As women age, their androgen levels may increase while their estrogen levels may decrease. For men, the opposite happens—they experience an increase in estrogen levels and a reduction in testosterone levels. These changes cause dryness of the skin, which speeds up the aging process. Certain supplements may help balance testosterone levels, but you should consult with your doctor first before taking any supplementation.

Chapter 5: Hormones and Your Diet

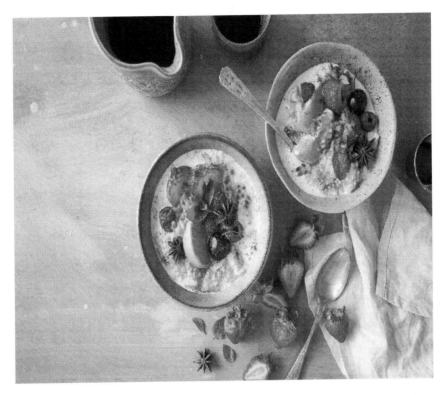

Changes in hormonal levels affect all men and women throughout their lives. The thing is, these changes affect each individual differently. When it comes to maintaining the health and balance of your hormones, your diet plays a vital role. You may have noticed that most of the suggested natural remedies always require you to follow a healthy and balanced diet. The reason is that foods can either have positive or negative effects on your body's hormone production.

Here is a quick rundown of the importance of different types of foods on your hormones:

Vegetables rich in antioxidants promote hormonal balance

No matter what diet you plan to follow, it should always include antioxidant-rich vegetables. Antioxidants are essential for the health of the body—and hormones—because of their anti-aging and protective characteristics. Some examples of dark green vegetables are spinach, asparagus, broccoli, kale, etc. The brightly colored vegetables that you should eat include carrots, bell peppers, onions, and many more. The starchy varieties include beets, squash, sweet potatoes, etc.

Fats promote hormonal balance

Healthy fats are a crucial component of hormonal balance. In particular, omega-3 and omega-6 are essential for the production of hormones and for maintaining the proper functions of hormones. The body needs fats to stabilize hormones and rebuild cells, especially for the reproductive system of women. You can get healthy fats from egg yolks, nuts, seeds, avocados, fatty fish, etc.

Spices and herbs help the body heal

Apart from containing antioxidants, most herbs and spices promote healing, which is why you should include them in your diet as well. Some examples of healing herbs and spices include ginger, turmeric, cumin, cayenne, cinnamon, garlic, and many more.

Of course, lean proteins and healthy carbs should also be part of your diet. Following a healthy and well-balanced diet provides your body with the essential nutrients to ensure overall health and hormonal balance. But if you are suffering from hormonal imbalances, specific diets may be more beneficial for you.

The Alkaline Diet and Hormonal Health

Even though you do not realize it, hormones have a significant effect on your life all day, every day. They have an effect on our appetite, digestion, libido, fertility, moods, mental clarity, weight, etc. When it comes to the health of your hormones, you should follow a balanced, nutrient-rich diet that focuses on whole foods. Such foods can help you achieve the right pH levels in your body, which maintains your hormonal balance.

Ideally, your blood pH level should be slightly alkaline. If you want your hormones to function at their best, you should try to maintain a pH level of 7.2 to 7.4 each day. To do this, you may want to follow the alkaline diet.

While on this diet, 60% of the calories you consume would come from alkaline-forming foods, while 40% can come from acid-forming foods. When choosing the latter, opt for healthier varieties. Following the alkaline diet does not mean that you should eliminate acid-forming foods. After all, healthy types of these foods, such as organic and lean animal protein, are essential for hormone building. While on the alkaline diet, though, you should be more aware of what you are eating. At each meal, top up your plate with healthy, alkaline-forming foods to maintain the slightly alkaline pH level that your body needs.

Apart from potentially improving the balance of the pH levels of the body, proponents of this diet claim that it also helps fight disease and promote weight loss. Some research even suggests that the alkaline diet can be especially beneficial for people suffering from kidney disease (Passey, 2016). The main reason is that it encourages you to consume more vegetables and fruits while limiting your intake of high-fat dairy and processed meat products.

While there is no evidence proving that the alkaline diet can change the pH levels of the body, the diet can improve your health. Some of the best types of alkaline-forming foods to eat to promote hormonal health and balance include:

- Coconut oil
- Avocados
- Wild-caught, organic salmon
- Kale
- Spinach
- Collards
- Broccoli
- Brussels sprouts
- Cauliflower
- Cabbage
- Quinoa
- Red bell peppers
- Sweet potatoes
- Flax seeds
- Chickpeas
- Cucumbers
- Sprouts
- Buckwheat

The Anti-Inflammatory Diet and Hormonal Health

In recent years, different kinds of anti-inflammatory diets have gained a lot of popularity and for a good reason. Anti-inflammatory diets encourage the consumption of fresh foods and foods that are high in healthy fats. These diets also allow you to consume red wine and nuts in moderation while staying away from red meat as much as possible. Anti-inflammatory foods promote the health of the hormones because they focus on a healthy and nutritionally-sound approach to eating.

Since you will be staying away from foods that cause inflammation, following an anti-inflammatory diet may also promote hormonal balance. Also, the foods you would eat while on this diet contain a lot of antioxidants that protect the body against inflammation and its harmful effects. Here are more pointers for you for following an anti-inflammatory diet:

Limit or eliminate foods that cause inflammation

For a lot of people, foods like soy, gluten, alcohol, processed dairy, processed snacks, processed meats, and sugar can trigger inflammation. When this happens, it causes imbalances in your hormonal levels. For this tip, you may have to do trial and error to determine which foods cause inflammation and which foods do not. When you discover the foods that do cause inflammation in your body, try to limit your consumption of these.

Consume a minimum of 3 cups of veggies each day

Vegetables are rich in phytonutrients (plant hormones) that promote hormonal balance. They also give you fiber to improve digestion and elimination of toxins, thus leading to an improvement in your overall equilibrium. Vegetables also contain prebiotic fibers that are essential for the good bacteria in the gut. If you're not used to eating vegetables, you can start with minimal amounts each day and gradually add more, allowing your body to adjust to the added fiber intake.

Include adaptogens in your diet

Certain adaptogenic herbs such as Rhodiola, maca, and ashwagandha can help with stress adaptation. Adaptogens can improve your body's overall stress-resistance, not just a specific system or organ. This, in turn, may help bring balance and harmony to your hormonal levels while reducing inflammation as well.

Focus on foods that contain healthy fats

As much as possible, try to avoid oils that contain high quantities of omega-6, such as canola oil, sunflower oil, shortenings, peanut oil, and the likes. Instead, focus on healthy fats and oils, such as fatty fish, algae oil, walnuts, chia seeds, avocados, coconut oil, etc.

Limit your caffeine intake

When you consume too much caffeine, this slows your thyroid down while increasing your cortisol levels. It may also aggravate existing gut disorders like acid reflux. While it is okay to consume 1 to 2 cups of coffee each day, try not to drink excessive amounts of caffeinated beverages like coffee, tea, and the like. But if you are trying hard to fix hormonal imbalances and lower your inflammation levels, then you may want to avoid caffeine until you achieve your desired results.

Consider going off your birth control (for women)

Unless you are taking birth control pills out of necessity, you may want to wean yourself off this hormonal method. Since birth control pills contain synthetic hormones, they may hurt your digestion, natural hormones, and thyroid function. However, you shouldn't just quit cold-turkey. Do this gradually so that your body gets the chance to adjust, stabilize, and bring back balance to itself.

Mindful Eating and Hormonal Health

Have you ever heard of mindful eating?

This is a new trend in the wellness and nutrition world, and it can help improve your hormonal health. Even though mindful eating may seem unfamiliar to you, mindfulness is a concept that you may have already heard about, primarily if you practice yoga and meditation. Simply put, mindfulness is a practice of being aware and present at each moment. When you practice mindfulness, you will focus all of your mental energy on what you are experiencing at that very moment. You allow your experiences and feelings to overcome you and accepting everything as it is. Nowadays, researchers are looking into the different types of mindfulness practices that can help with the management of stress, pain, anxiety, and even a negative relationship with food. Having such a relationship with food leads to poor eating habits like emotional eating, binge eating, and other types of eating pattern issues.

Mindful eating involves eating with attention and intention. This helps increase your awareness of the food you are eating, improve your relationship with food, and boost digestive processes. Before going through some tips for mindful eating, let's take a look at the different benefits of this practice:

Your body will be able to absorb nutrients more effectively

Since your food will be digested more efficiently, your body can absorb the nutrients from your food better, too. This means that your hormones, organs, and cells get more nutrients, so they can continue functioning at their best.

You may experience less gas, bloating, and other similar issues

When you take the time to consume your meals by chewing each mouthful carefully before swallowing, this makes it easier to digest your food properly. In turn, it reduces the amount of undigested food but gets fermented and causing you to bloat. Mindful eating also helps reduce acid reflux, constipation, diarrhea, and other digestive problems.

It helps reduce your stress levels

Mindful eating helps lower your cortisol levels naturally. This, in turn, improves your mood, concentration, anxiety, sleep, memory, PMS symptoms, etc.

You will gain a healthy and positive relationship with food

If you are an emotional eater, mindful eating can help you overcome this. As you eat more mindfully, this changes your relationship with food into something healthier. You will be in control of what you eat and how much you eat. With this improvement, you will also learn how to appreciate and enjoy the food you eat more as well.

You may even lose weight

Mindful eating makes you feel full and prevent you to eat less. You can know whether you are still hungry or can stop eating. Thus, you will only eat the right amount of food at each meal. Over time, you may notice that you are losing weight.

Mindful eating helps you disengage from your self-defeating and habitual eating behaviors and replace them with more supportive and skillful actions. The more you practice mindfulness in eating, the more you will notice a decrease in emotional eating, food cravings, symptoms of eating disorders, binge eating, and psychological stress caused by our poor eating habits.

Apart from all the health benefits, mindful eating can also help you enjoy the entire eating experience with restraint and moderation. Pair these mindful eating practices with the alkaline diet, the anti-inflammatory diet, or any other kind of diet that promotes the health of the hormones, this gives you a recipe for success. Here are some tips to guide you as you practice eating mindfully:

Reflect upon your feelings

Even before you start your meal, take a moment to reflect. Do you feel hungry? Sad? Happy? Bored? Stressed? What do you need? What do you want? After taking a moment to reflect, you will become more aware of your feelings. Then, you can determine whether you really want to eat, what you would like to eat at that moment, and how you would like to eat your meal.

After taking some time to reflect, take another moment to be grateful for what you are about to eat. Acknowledge, appreciate, and be thankful for all the labor that went into your meal. This will give you a richer appreciation as you are eating the food on your plate.

Sit down to eat

It's never a good idea to eat while on-the-go. Mindful eating does not work that way. Instead, you should take a seat and focus on your meal. This helps you appreciate more what you are eating and keep track of the amount of food you have already eaten.

Eat appropriate portions

You shouldn't be eating the food right out of the box, bag, or container. This leads to overeating and prevents you from fully appreciating the food you are eating because you can't see it.

You may also consider using a smaller plate. If you see less food, you may crave less. Using small plates allows you to control your portions. This is an especially good strategy if you go to eat-all-you-can buffets.

Eliminate any distractions while you are eating

When you eat while watching television or browsing on your phone, you won't be able to notice how much you have eaten, what the food tasted like, and if you chewed your food properly before swallowing.

Talking is another distraction that can take you away from mindful eating. Once in a while, try to consume your meals in silence. Allow your mind to wander, accept the thoughts you have, and gently guide your mind back to your eating experience.

Put down your utensils in between bites

Usually, you would already be setting up your next bite using your utensils while you are still chewing your previous bite. But if you want to be more mindful when eating, it's better to put your utensils down until you have chewed and swallowed the food inside your mouth. Only then should you pick up the utensils again for the next bite. This slows down your eating process and helps you become more mindful.

Chew each bite 30 times

Ideally, you should try to get 30 chews out of each bite you eat, depending on the texture of the food. Doing so allows you to enjoy the flavors before swallowing and helps prevent overeating because your gut has time to send a message to your brain that you're already full.

Remember that you do not have to clean your plate all the time

Most children are taught to finish everything on their plates before leaving the table. Now that you are an adult, you may still be doing this, forcing yourself to eat everything even though you are already full. If so, it's time to break this habit. Once you feel full, you can pack up your leftovers and eat them for your next meal or the next time you're feeling hungry.

All of these tips can help you become more aware of all the aspects of your food—from the tastes, flavors, textures, smells, etc. This makes your eating experience richer, allowing you to appreciate each meal fully. The better you get at mindful eating, the more you will start experiencing the health benefits this practice has to offer.

Taking Natural Supplements for Hormonal Health

Hormone imbalances can impact your physical and mental health. Any hormonal shifts can cause noticeable changes in your body, your feelings, your cognitive ability, and even the development of several medical conditions. Apart from your diet, another effective way to bring back your hormonal balance is by taking natural supplements. Such supplements can regulate and support your hormones, thus reducing some of the adverse symptoms of these imbalances. Some of the best supplements to take are:

B-Complex

B-vitamins are essential for your health. Having a deficiency in these vitamins can cause fatigue and low energy since they are crucial for metabolic functions. In particular, B6 is essential to boost the production of progesterone. Vitamin B6 also supports corpus luteum development, gives the immune system a boost, and works with the enzymes of the liver to eliminate excess estrogen.

Calcium

Taking calcium supplements can improve bone density. Supplementing your body with calcium is essential, especially as you age since it reduces the risk of breaking your bones when you fall over or get into accidents.

Copper

Taking copper supplements may reduce your risk of getting depressed as it may help improve your mood. Also, it can reverse the enlargement of the heart due to pressure overload.

Magnesium and Vitamin B6

Taking magnesium supplements can reduce inflammation, ease the effects of stress, normalize heart rhythms, lower blood pressure, and improve sleep. When you take this mineral together with vitamin B6, it can help reduce anxiety and stress. For women, this combination improves the severe symptoms of PMS.

Niacin

Also known as vitamin B3, this vitamin helps you feel more relaxed and allows you to sleep more restfully. The reason is that vitamin B3 relaxes your muscle tissues, thus boosting blood circulation. Because of the effects of this vitamin, it can reduce depression, anxiety, and stress. However, one side effect of niacin is skin flushing; therefore, you must consult with your doctor first before you start taking niacin supplementation.

Omega-3

The hormones of the body are created out of omega-3s. This is why this type of supplement is highly recommended for people who suffer from hormone disorders. Also, omega-3s can decrease inflammatory damage that may interfere with your hormonal balance.

Probiotics

Hormonal balance is linked with the health of your gut. Since probiotics feed the healthy bacteria in your gut, this may lead to an improvement in the production of certain hormones. If you do not want to take probiotic supplements, you may include foods that are rich in probiotics in your diet.

Vitamin C

Taking vitamin C supplements can help lower your adrenaline and cortisol levels. They also help lower inflammation, boost immune function, and reduce oxidative stress. For women, vitamin C is essential for fertility. Women who have fertility issues but aren't responding to other medications or supplements may take vitamin C to help restore their fertility.

Vitamin D

This vitamin plays a part in the regulation of the thyroid hormone and insulin. When you are deficient in vitamin D, you may be at risk for thyroid antibodies or autoimmune thyroid disorders. Taking vitamin D supplements can balance your blood sugar levels and regulate your insulin flow. This, in turn, allows the natural hormone cycles of the body to work more effectively.

Zinc

Taking zinc supplements may enhance the emotional status and brain function, particularly in premenopausal women. This supplement can also give your mood a boost so that you do not end up feeling depressed. Another benefit of zinc is that it may help improve your resilience against stress while improving bone mass too.

Other Tips, Strategies, and Healthy Dietary Practices for Hormonal Health

If you discover that you are suffering from hormonal imbalance, you are not alone. As much as we would like to maintain hormonal health and balance, there are just so many factors that can mess things up. Do not believe those who claim that there is nothing you can do to restore hormonal balance. In fact, it's the exact opposite. Being aware of your hormones and how they affect your life is important as this will help you take the necessary steps to keep your hormones healthy.

Hormonal health and balance require stable levels of blood sugar, healthy digestion, well-functioning liver, and a healthy endocrine system. To wrap up this chapter about hormones and your diet, let's go through other tips, strategies, and healthy dietary practices for you to start doing now. All of these can help you improve your hormonal health and boost your overall health too!

Take a shot to start your day right

In order to activate your digestion in the morning, you may want to try taking a shot of water mixed with apple cider vinegar. Simply combine a tablespoon of vinegar with three tablespoons of water, mix well, and take that shot! Apple cider vinegar improves the gut microbiome, and it also helps the body metabolize fat. Just make sure to choose a brand of apple cider vinegar that is organic and raw.

Have a warming tonic

After taking your first shot of a day, it's time to wake up your mind and further stimulate your digestive system by drinking a warming tonic. You may try lemon tea to stimulate your digestive system. You may also try ginger tea that has the same effect and even provides anti-inflammatory benefits.

Follow a healthy and balanced diet

This tip has been mentioned time and time again because it is extremely important, and it cannot be emphasized enough. As you plan or choose your meals, make sure that you include different whole foods, plant-based options, and other healthy food options that provide the nutrients that you need to keep your endocrine system healthy. Opt for fresh, real foods instead of processed ones that may do more harm than good, especially in terms of your hormones.

Make sure that you are getting enough protein

This is extremely important for the health of your hormones. In particular, dietary protein provides you with essential amino acids that your body cannot produce on its own. These amino acids help maintain bone, skin, and muscle health. Protein also affects the release of hormones that regulate food intake and appetite. Eating enough protein helps decrease your ghrelin levels while stimulating the production of hormones that make you feel full.

Limit your consumption of junk food, sugar, refined carbs, and dairy

All these foods tend to wreak havoc on your entire endocrine system. They may weaken your adrenal glands, liver, and blood, thus leading to inadequate hormonal function. Excessive amounts of caffeine and sugar cause spikes in your insulin levels, while processed foods increase the number of damaging free-radicals in your body. When you eat unhealthy foods like these, expect to have imbalanced hormones as well.

If you love dairy, you may feel disappointed to discover that this food group is also a no-no when it comes to hormonal health. Unfortunately, dairy products contain several types of natural hormones that shouldn't be combined with your hormones. If you can't stop yourself from consuming dairy, you should at least try to limit your consumption.

Avoid undereating and overeating

When you eat too little or too much—or do both irregularly—this may cause hormonal shifts in your body along with weight issues. Undereating or restricting your caloric intake too much tends to increase your body's production of cortisol. This, in turn, may promote weight gain. Also, some people who follow low-calorie diets may experience insulin resistance because of it.

Conversely, overeating reduces your insulin sensitivity while increasing your levels of insulin. Of course, overeating constantly may result in being overweight or obese—two conditions that lead to a host of other health issues. When it comes to eating, make sure that you only consume enough to maintain a healthy weight and a healthy hormonal balance.

Apart from the two diets discussed in the previous section, you may also want to consider other types of diets that can potentially improve your hormonal health. Some examples of these diets are:

Grain-free

Gluten is the primary protein found in wheat. Recently, gluten has gotten a bad reputation—mainly because it's not good for the health of your hormones. Therefore, going grain-free may be a good option for you. Replacing grains with healthy proteins, fats, and phytonutrient-rich carbs may improve your hormonal health. However, if you eliminate grains from your diet right away, this might result in struggles with binge eating, food craving, and other eating habits that will wreak havoc on your hormones. If you want to follow this diet, you should start slow so that your body does not get shocked and you do not end up feeling miserable about the diet.

Intermittent Fasting

Along with keto, this is one of the trendiest diets now. While it does not restrict any kind of foods or food groups, intermittent fasting involves going for intermediate or short periods of time without eating anything. You have "fasting periods" and "feasting periods" throughout the day depending on the schedule you have chosen.

This diet may help stabilize your levels of blood sugar and promote weight loss, both of which are good for your hormones. However, this diet may cause hormone disruption in women. Therefore, women should speak with their doctors first before following intermittent fasting. Come up with a plan for how to follow this eating pattern while still ensuring the health and balance of your hormones.

Ketogenic Diet

This is a low-carb, high-fat diet that allows you to consume moderate amounts of protein. The main goal of the ketogenic diet is to force your body into a state of ketosis. While in this state, your body starts burning fat for fuel instead of glucose. One of the main and most appealing health benefits of this diet is weight loss. However, this is also considered a highly specialized diet. Therefore, if you plan to go keto, speak with your doctor first. You should have trusted medical support to guide you as you follow the diet.

Raw Vegan

Vegetables and fruits of different colors—whether you eat them raw or cooked—are beneficial for the health of your hormones. But when following the raw vegan diet, you should only consume plant-based food sources that have been heated below 104°F. The good part is that you won't be eating processed, refined, or pasteurized foods. However, the downside of this diet is that it may compromise your gut health, especially if you're not used to eating fruits and vegetables in their raw or semi-cooked form.

The bottom line is this: when it comes to ensuring the health and balance of your hormones through your diet, listening to your body is key. There is no point in following a diet or taking natural supplements when it causes adverse side effects. We all have different bodies and different hormonal balances. What may work for some people might not work for others. Customization is important along with communicating openly with your doctor to ensure your health and safety.

Chapter 6: The Importance of
Hormonal Balance

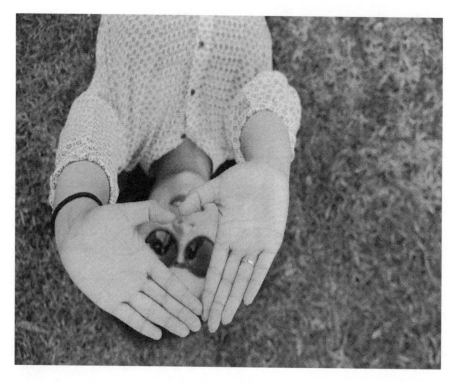

Hormones are crucial to maintaining the proper functioning of the body. Therefore, when you experience any hormonal imbalance, this may lead to several health issues. As substances of the body, hormones are particularly powerful. Even when your blood has low concentrations of these hormones, it can affect the target organs and systems significantly. Whenever hormones are secreted, they do not last for such a long time in the blood. Instead, they usually last between a few seconds to half an hour. Some hormones produce immediate effects on the body, while others may take a few hours or even a few days before you may feel their effects.

Throughout your life, the hormonal concentration in your blood varies continuously. Each of the hormones must be individually and regulated explicitly to fulfill the needs of your body. They must work in perfect balance as most of them interact with each other and with the other vital substances within the body.

When one or more of your hormones are secreted in excessive or abnormal amounts, this causes a hormonal disruption or a hormonal imbalance. Since each of the hormones produces its own effects on the body, the consequences depend on the gland or hormone affected, as well as the intensity and nature of the hormonal imbalance. As previously mentioned, there are specific points throughout a person's life where you would naturally experience hormonal imbalances, including puberty, menopause, pregnancy, and so on. These imbalances occur, along with the changes in the body. In some cases, hormonal imbalances can also be caused by disease or aging.

In both men and women, hormonal imbalances occur at varying ages and for several reasons. Because of this, it is quite challenging to determine the risk factors for these imbalances. What doctors know for sure is that there are certain groups of people who have a higher risk for hormonal imbalances—to be precise, those who are at certain stages of their lives. When you suffer from hormonal imbalances, you may experience many symptoms depending on which of your hormones are imbalanced, which gland is affected, and other reasons. The most common symptoms of hormonal imbalances are:

- Unexplained weight gain
- Unexplained weight loss
- Fatigue
- Vaginal dryness
- Hot flashes
- Reduced libido
- Erectile dysfunction
- Cold intolerance
- Constipation

Depending on the severity of your condition, the symptoms you experience could be much more than this. Often, a combination of the typical symptoms of a specific disorder allows a doctor to make the proper diagnosis for your hormonal imbalance. Because of all the adverse side effects that hormonal imbalances may cause, maintaining the appropriate balance of your hormones is of the utmost importance.

Natural Ways to Restore Your Hormonal Balance

Hormonal imbalances can have a significant impact on your appetite, mood, sex drive, and all the other aspects of your health. Some factors are beyond your control, such as aging and going through the normal stages of life. However, there are manageable factors (diet, stress levels, etc.) that can also have an impact on your hormonal balance.

Hormones are produced and secreted by the endocrine system. If any of the glands that are part of this system are affected by illness, this can cause a ripple effect, thus making you feel different symptoms. Worse, it may lead to chronic diseases over time.

Fortunately, there are several ways for you to restore hormonal balance. These include:

Make sure that you get enough sleep

While sleep is essential for women in order to bring back their regular periods, it matters for men, too. Clocking in enough hours of sleep each night can help restore hormonal balance. In fact, this is probably the most crucial factor that would ensure a hormonal balance. Throughout the day, your hormonal levels may fluctuate in response to specific issues, such as the quality of your sleep. If you always lack adequate sleep, you may experience some adverse effects like:

- Appetite issues

- Diabetes

- Weight gain, leading to obesity

On the other hand, getting a full night's sleep each night without interruption allows your body to regulate its hormonal levels.

Move for your health

We have already discussed the importance of exercise and physical activity for the health of the hormones. Making movement part of your life can also help restore your hormonal balance. This, in turn, helps improve your memory, sexual function, sleep, digestion, and other issues that you may have experienced because of hormonal imbalances.

Learn how to avoid toxicity

Each day, our bodies get exposed to chemicals from all around us. There are chemicals in the air, various health and wellness products, our food, and others that disrupt the endocrine system and the hormones they produce. To deal with this issue, it's recommended to read the labels of all the products you purchase to find out what they really contain. You may also opt for a detoxification program to cleanse your body of these harmful toxins.

Manage your stress effectively

Chronic stress is awful for your hormonal balance. If you do not have an imbalance, stress may cause it. If you already have an existing hormonal imbalance, stress may aggravate your condition. Deep breathing exercises, yoga, and other relaxing activities can help reduce your stress levels. Also, learning how to eliminate or manage your stressors more effectively can help bring balance to your hormonal levels.

Enjoy a cup of green tea

Generally speaking, green tea is one of the healthiest beverages out there (apart from water). It contains antioxidants and other compounds that improve your metabolic health. Green tea can lower your fasting insulin levels as well as aid in the management of oxidative stress.

Eliminate or avoid smoking and excessive alcohol consumption

Tobacco smoke can also disrupt your hormonal levels. Researchers have discovered that this smoke can alter the levels of thyroid hormones, stimulate the production of pituitary hormones, and elevate the levels of cortisol and other steroid hormones (Darbre, 2018).

While drinking small amounts of alcohol isn't harmful to your health, consuming more than this may start disturbing hormonal levels, particularly in young men. Therefore, if you have any concerns with hormonal imbalances, you may want to eliminate or even limit your alcohol consumption.

Have regular check-ups with your doctor

One of the best ways to maintain hormonal balance is to have your hormone levels checked regularly. If you are feeling any odd symptoms and you cannot pinpoint the cause, you may be suffering from one kind of hormonal imbalance or another. Have yourself checked so that your doctor can come up with a proper diagnosis. Once you are diagnosed with a hormonal imbalance, you will be able to take the necessary steps in order to restore balance and improve your health.

The Best Foods to Restore Hormonal Balance

The foods that you eat can have a significant impact on hormonal balance and health. While people seldom think of foods as a remedy to treat various conditions, when it comes to hormonal balance, certain types of food can help. Including these healthy options to your diet may restore the balance of your hormonal levels while improving your overall health. That way, you won't have to take medications to improve your condition, as these may cause several adverse side effects. If you want to restore hormonal balance, here are some foods you should pile on your plate:

Avocados

Apart from being a delicious addition to any dish or meal, avocados are incredibly healthy fruits. Consuming this fruit can help with the regulation of your stress hormones and menstrual cycle (for women). After all, avocados contain plant sterols that have a positive effect on progesterone and estrogen. Avocados are also rich in beta-sitosterol, a compound that has positive effects on blood cholesterol levels.

Broccoli

Remember when your parents kept reminding you to eat the broccoli on your plate? If you listened then and you still eat this green veggie now, good for you! Apart from all the health benefits broccoli offers, it also helps bring balance to your hormonal levels. In particular, it promotes estrogen metabolism by eliminating "bad" estrogens in the body that come from the environment.

Eggs

Eggs contain the vitamin choline that helps the body with acetylcholine production. This is a type of neurotransmitter that is crucial for brain health, the nervous system, development, and memory. Eggs are also rich in omega-3 fatty acids that support the health and functions of the brain. With a healthy nervous system and brain, you will be able to deal with stress more effectively, which helps restore your hormonal balance.

Flax seeds

These seeds are rich in beneficial omega-3 fatty acids. They also contain phytoestrogens, plant-based compounds that can mimic estrogen, bind to the body's estrogen receptors, and help the body with excess estrogen excretion. These seeds can prevent or improve other hormonal issues like menopausal symptoms, osteoporosis, etc.

Kale

This green, leafy vegetable is rich in fiber, making it ideal for the health of your gut. When your gut is healthy, this helps encourage hormonal balance. Fiber is also beneficial for your insulin sensitivity while making you feel full for more extended periods. Kale is also rich in magnesium, a mineral that supports healthy testosterone and estrogen levels.

Nuts

Different types of nuts can affect your endocrine system mainly by helping to decrease your cholesterol levels. Consuming nuts can reduce your insulin levels while maintaining healthy levels of blood sugar. In particular, walnuts contain polyphenols, a type of compound that protects your cardiovascular system from damage caused by free radicals. This compound also has anti-inflammatory characteristics to help prevent a hormonal imbalance.

Pomegranate

This fruit is rich in antioxidants, beneficial compounds that help prevent the production of excess estrogen. It contains a natural compound that inhibits the conversion of estrone into estradiol, a dominant type of estrogen that plays a role in the development of cancers that depend on hormones. Because of this particular benefit, some researchers claim that pomegranate can potentially prevent some types of breast cancer, especially the ones that respond to estrogen (American Association for Cancer Research, 2010).

Quinoa

With all the health benefits quinoa has to offer, it's widely considered a superfood. It contains fiber, protein, and a wide range of minerals. Consuming quinoa can help regulate your bowel movement by improving your digestion. It is also rich in zinc, a mineral that helps with the production of the thyroid hormone.

Tempeh

Soy is one type of food that is controversial for several reasons. But choosing good soy sources such as organic tempeh can provide you with positive benefits, mainly from the isoflavones content of soy. Fermented soy products such as tempeh and miso can provide probiotics that boost your mood and digestion.

Wild Salmon

This fatty fish contains a specific protein that brings balance to your hunger hormones while increasing the feeling of fullness. Salmon also contains omega-3s that help with the synthesis of hormones responsible for regulating inflammation, blood clotting, and arterial function.

Your diet is an essential aspect of your health. The healthier your food choices are, the healthier you will become. As much as possible, try to stay away from processed, packaged, or pre-prepared foods. Instead, opt for whole foods and natural food sources. These may help promote hormonal balance to avoid any health issues.

Chapter 7: How Does Hormonal Balance Affect Your Metabolism?

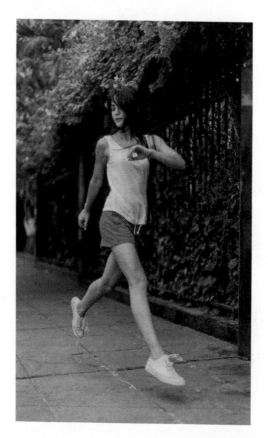

Achieving and maintaining a healthy weight is a common concern for both men and women. For a lot of people, weight management is a struggle that gets even more difficult as they age. Now that you know how much hormones affect different aspects of your body, you should know that it also affects your metabolism. When it comes to metabolism, here are the glands that are most involved, along with the hormones that they produce:

Adrenal Glands

The adrenal glands produce hormones that enable the body to adapt to situations that are either dysfunctionally or functionally changing. These hormones are essential because they determine how your body accesses fuel and how it utilizes that fuel from the food you eat. They help determine whether your body uses this fuel as energy or stores it as fats.

Adrenal glands also secrete stress hormones that are responsible for the regulation of glucose from your muscle and liver cells. This secretion either slows down or speeds up the metabolic rate of your body. These processes are nutrient-dependent, meaning they depend on the food you eat. Therefore, when you consume the right foods, especially when you are faced with stressful situations, your body will utilize the fuel instead of storing it.

Pituitary Gland

This gland produces hormones that control the actions of the other hormones within your body. Therefore, it also influences your metabolism. As long as everything is running smoothly, your pituitary gland runs smoothly. Specifically, if any of the other glands or hormones that are responsible for your metabolism are "out of whack," the pituitary gland helps bring back the balance. But if your pituitary gland is affected, then you may experience several adverse effects on your metabolism and your overall health.

Thyroid Gland

This gland is considered a metabolic superstar. You can think of it as the furnace of your body. In this analogy, the thyroid gland itself is the thermostat, the hypothalamus is the person who controls the thermostat, and the hormones produced by the gland—T3 and T4—provide the heat. When your thyroid gland and hypothalamus aren't working correctly, this will affect your metabolism. The hormones produced by the thyroid gland have a direct influence on your metabolism through caloric and oxygen conversion.

Between the two hormones, T3 is much more potent than T4. But if you possess a hormone known as reverse T3 (RT3), this may block the healthy functioning of your thyroid gland. Although the hormone won't really "mess up" your weight loss goals, overproduction can significantly slow down your metabolic rate. When this happens, your body will stop burning fuel and start storing it instead.

When it comes to metabolism, the liver is essential, too. There are more than 600 metabolic functions that happen through the liver, and these are only the ones we know about. Virtually every hormone, nutrient, and chemical must be activated by the liver. While technically not a gland, when hormones are secreted by the different glands of the endocrine system, your liver breaks the hormones down to make them biologically active so that they can start doing their work.

The liver influences swelling, water weight, electrolyte balance, and dehydration. It is responsible for the conversion of B-vitamins into co-enzymes and metabolism of macronutrients (fats, carbohydrates, and proteins). The liver also produces carnitine, which transmits fat to the mitochondria and cells—a process that influences 90% of your metabolism. The faster your liver can produce carnitine, the more efficient your metabolism becomes.

Your metabolism and hormones are intertwined profoundly. Metabolism isn't as simple as the rate at which your body burns calories. Instead, it involves all the processes of how your body utilizes energy and stores energy from the food you eat. Apart from burning calories, metabolism also converts carbohydrates, proteins, and fats into glucose, fatty acids, amino acids, and other compounds then transport these into your body's cells. It also involves the growth and maintenance of muscles as well as the process of breaking down the body's fat stores.

And all of these metabolic processes are controlled and regulated by the hormones. Therefore, to ensure the smooth operation of the body's systems, hormonal balance is crucial. If any of your hormonal levels go up too high or go down too low, this may throw your metabolism off balance as well.

Hormonal Balance and Weight Loss

Hormones are powerful chemical substances in the body that are considered as "messengers." As with so many other aspects of your life, hormonal balance can affect weight loss because hormones regulate your metabolism. Losing weight through fat loss can be achieved through your hormones. Specifically, these hormones are:

Cortisol

This stress hormone is closely connected to insulin, another hormone that affects weight loss. If your cortisol levels go up because of stress, your levels of insulin go up too. This, in turn, makes it very difficult to lose weight. Stress can also cause weight-loss resistance. In fact, science proves that you can "think yourself thin."

On the other hand, when you have stressful thoughts—including stressful thoughts about how much you weigh—these tend to stimulate metabolic ideas that cause insulin resistance and weight gain. Therefore, if you want to improve your stress responses and balance your cortisol levels to promote weight loss, here are some tips:

- Take the time to improve your social life. This goes a long way to making you feel happier and more positive, thus reducing your stress levels.

- Actively seek activities that promote relaxation and do them!

- Change your negative, stressful thoughts into positive ones. Try to consciously think of happy thoughts that will bring you closer to your weight-loss goals.

Glucagon

This hormone provides the opposite effect of insulin. Therefore, when your insulin levels go up, your glucagon levels go down. Glucagon is essential for weight loss because it is a fat-burning hormone and secreted when you consume protein. Therefore, if you want more of this hormone in your bloodstream, make sure that you consume glucagon-stimulating foods at each meal such as lean meat, eggs, turkey, chicken, fish, yogurt, cottage cheese, etc.

Insulin

The primary function of this hormone is to regulate glucose levels and fat storage. Therefore, when you consume a lot of foods that promote insulin secretion (e.g., refined sugars and flours), you may experience insulin spikes. When this happens, weight loss becomes tough. Instead of consuming such foods, opt for foods that contain essential fatty acids as these may promote weight loss.

Sex Hormones

Imbalances concerning your sex hormones may also cause issues with your weight. For both men and women, excess levels of estrogen may cause weight gain. And when you eat a lot of refined carbs and sugary foods, or you consume a lot of alcohol, these cause spikes in your estrogen levels. In men, low levels of testosterone may cause them to gain fat and lose muscle apart from other adverse effects. Here are some tips to improve and balance your levels of sex hormones for weight loss:

- Consume foods that are rich in fibers, especially organic fruits and vegetables.

- Find the right types of exercise for your own body to build muscle and lose fat.

- Limit or eliminate alcohol consumption.

Thyroid Hormones

Since the thyroid gland plays a vital role in metabolism, this means that the thyroid hormones also play an essential role in reaching and maintaining a healthy weight. In fact, when you have a hypothyroid, you may suffer from weight-loss resistance. To help improve your thyroid hormones to lose weight, here are some tips:

- Follow a balanced diet to ensure the health of your thyroid gland.

- Take supplements that promote the health of your thyroid gland as needed.

- Have your thyroid functions and hormone levels tested regularly. Request your doctor to check the levels of your thyroid-stimulating hormone, free T3, free T4, and even your thyroid antibodies and anti-thyroglobulin antibodies.

- Consider hormone replacement therapy for your thyroid hormones. Ask your doctor if you need to take such therapy.

The Role of Exercise in Hormonal and Metabolic Balance

Every time we have discussed tips and strategies to improve your hormonal health and balance, exercise is always part of the list. This is because exercise improves your overall health by promoting hormonal—and metabolic—balance. Did you know that some hormones are considered as "exercise hormones"? Here are these exercise hormones and the physiological functions they are responsible for:

Adrenaline and Noradrenaline

These hormones play a significant role in the production of energy as well as the regulation of bodily functions while you are performing cardiorespiratory exercises. Adrenaline increases your cardiac output, blood sugar, promotes glycogen breakdown to increase energy and supports the metabolism of fat. Noradrenaline performs similar functions while also narrowing the blood vessels of the body parts that aren't involved in your exercise routine.

Cortisol

When you exercise, this increases your body's levels of cortisol. This, in turn, increases your heart rate and blood pressure while releasing glucose into your bloodstream. However, when this occurs for an extended period, it starts wreaking havoc on your metabolism as it affects your other hormones too. This is why you shouldn't over-exercise or over-exert yourself in terms of exercise.

Estrogen

Although women need this hormone, excessive amounts of estrogen may lead to several health issues. When you exercise, this reverses the trend, thus lowering your risk of developing breast cancer and other illnesses.

Glucagon

The secretion of this hormone stimulates the flow of free fatty acids, as well as the increase in blood glucose. Both of these are crucial for providing fuel as you are exercising.

Human Growth Hormone

This is a fat-burning hormone that forces the body to use energy from your fat stores first. In particular, your body produces high levels of this hormone when performing plyometric exercises, strength training, and HIIT.

Insulin

If you have high levels of insulin, your body tends to store fat, especially in your tummy, hips, and thighs. Unfortunately, the more you gain weight, the more your body produces insulin. This creates a vicious cycle that you can bring to a stop by exercising regularly.

Insulin-Like Growth Factor

This peptide hormone supports the functions of the human growth hormone in terms of repairing protein damage caused by exercise. Because of this function, this hormone is essential for muscle growth.

Irisin

This is the actual "exercise hormone" as it combats fat in two ways. First, it triggers specific genes that transform white fat into brown fat. Second, it regulates the undifferentiated stem cells, so they contribute to bone-building rather than storing fat. This hormone is produced when you start sweating while exercising.

Testosterone

In both men and women, this hormone burns fat, increases energy, builds muscles, and strengthens the bones. To increase the levels of testosterone in men, the best type of exercise is strength training. For women, it's a combination of resistance training, cardiovascular conditioning, and HIIT.

Thyroid Hormone

Since this is the body's primary metabolic hormone, it is also vital for exercising. Regular workouts promote the function of this hormone, which improves metabolism so your body can burn fat faster.

Chapter 8: Hormone Fix

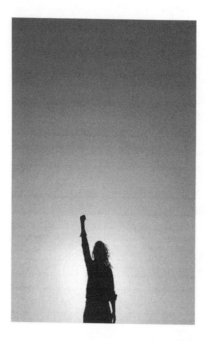

No matter how you look at it, hormones play an important role in your body and your life. Hormonal balance is crucial to the health of your body and mind. This is why "fixing your hormones" can improve your life in so many different ways. In this final chapter, let's take a look at some ways you can use the hormone fix to overcome some very common issues a lot of people experience.

Relieving Period Pain

All women have to experience menstrual periods for most of their lives. Unfortunately, for a lot of women, their periods may come with period pain as well. Women are especially prone to experiencing period pain when their hormones are imbalanced too. If you have imbalanced hormones, your period will likely come with pain and other symptoms as well. For this issue, here are some tips for your hormone fix:

Start "clean living" to calm your hormones

While most organic food items are significantly more expensive than the conventional options, base your choice on the health of your hormones. Those cheaper food options (such as processed foods) may contain toxins that will mess up your endocrine system. You may be saving a few dollars, you might be paying for this with your health.

Consider hormone therapy

Hormonal therapy and medication can help reduce your period pain and even regulate your menstrual cycle. Most women know this type of therapy as "birth control," and it is typically effective and safe for the purpose of balancing hormones, whether a woman is sexually active or not. Some options for hormone therapy include implants, the pill, skin patches, vaginal rings, IUD, etc. These can also make your periods shorter and lighter.

When it comes to hormone therapy, you may want to try other remedies first. If these natural remedies do not work, your doctor may recommend hormone therapy as a treatment option for the pain you feel during your period. The most commonly recommended option is the pill. This helps shorten periods and make them lighter while still maintaining the woman's normal cycle.

Apart from the mentioned hormone therapies, there are medications available for women who want to reduce pain and dysmenorrhea. However, these options tend to stop the occurrence of your monthly period or they may reduce the occurrence of your periods to once every couple of months.

There are different reasons why menstrual cramps and pain happen. If you experience these issues frequently, have yourself checked as there may be underlying issues like uterine fibroids, pelvic inflammatory disease or endometriosis. Learning the root cause of your problem can help your doctor determine the best treatment option for it.

Other remedies

Nowadays, doctors typically prescribe the pill for acne, erratic periods, and period pain. But if you are worried about the potential side effects of the pill, especially in terms of worsening your hormonal imbalance, you may first try natural remedies.

There are several herbal remedies that are useful as they provide gentle support to the natural levels of your hormones. However, if you are already using the pill, you should know that there are certain herbs that shouldn't be used in combination with it. One example of a natural herb that you can take is soy isoflavones (fermented). This time, it provides gentle support to your levels of oestrogen. Another natural option you can take is Agnus castus. This herb may gently support and bring balance to your levels of progesterone. Both of these herbs etc can help give you relief from period pain thus, making your period flow more smoothly and comfortably.

Improving the Quality of Sleep

When you are trying to improve your sleep quality, the last thing you would think about is your hormones. But when it comes to sleep and the hormones, they are dependent upon each other. When you get enough sleep, this gives your hormones time to replenish in order to function properly. Therefore, improving your quality of sleep is essential to improve your health and maintain your hormonal balance. For this issue, here are some tips for your hormone fix:

Perform relaxing activities right before going to bed

There are some hormones like cortisol and adrenaline that make it difficult for you to fall asleep at night. To combat the effects of these hormones or to reduce their production when it's almost time for you to go to bed, it's recommended to perform relaxing activities right before your bedtime. Try to come up with your own winding-down or bedtime routine that includes relaxing activities. This will help you fall asleep more easily.

Watch what you eat

When bedtime approaches, be careful of what you eat. For one, it's recommended to have a light dinner instead of a heavy one. Having heavy meals at night can cause a number of side effects that will keep you up all night. Also, avoid high-protein and high-fat foods during dinner. For beverages, stay away from those which contain caffeine or alcohol as these may disrupt your sleep.

Consider taking melatonin supplements or adaptogenic herbs

If sleep is really eluding you, consider taking melatonin supplements to help you sleep. However, you should only start with a low dose and you should only take these supplements for a short period of time. Adaptogenic herbs are also beneficial as they can help bring balance to your levels of cortisol. These herbs can also help your body adapt to different kinds of stress.

Turn off your electronic devices

While you might use these devices to "help you sleep," they actually have the opposite effect on you. These devices emit "blue light" that reduces your body's production of melatonin. If you really want to fall asleep on time, try to avoid using these devices right before going to bed.

If you have tried all of these strategies but you are still experiencing sleep difficulties, these might start having an adverse effect on your life. Consult a doctor who specializes in sleep disorders to help you improve your sleep quality. After all, your hormones are also working while you sleep. Here are some functions of the hormones related to sleep that you should be aware of:

- While you sleep, the growth hormone is released. This is essential for the growth and repair of tissues.
- Sleep helps balance your leptin and ghrelin levels in order to regulate your appetite.
- Not getting enough sleep might lower your prolactin levels which, in turn, weakens your immune system.
- The hormones cortisol and oxytocin are important as well since they influence our dreams.
- One great thing about balanced hormones is that they prevent you from having the urge to go to the toilet while sleeping. This benefit comes from the anti-diuretic and aldosterone hormones.

As you can see, hormones and sleep are linked with each other—and the health of one depends on the health of the other. That's why it's important for you to ensure that you get enough sleep each night.

Toning Up Your Body

One of the most effective things you can do to bring balance to your hormones is exercise. Exercising to ensure the health of your hormones will also help enhance your quality of life and tone your body up. Nowadays, most of us have resigned to living a sedentary lifestyle, especially for those who have desk jobs where they spend most of their time sitting in front of computers. Exercising regularly affects a number of hormones in different ways such as:

Boosts testosterone in men and estrogen in women

As men age, their levels of testosterone decrease naturally. But for men who exercise regularly, this boosts testosterone levels in order to slow down the natural effects caused by aging. Exercise is also beneficial for women as it boosts the levels of estrogen too. This helps minimize the menopause symptoms felt by women.

Releases serotonin

Physical activity and exercise help release serotonin, an important hormone that promotes restful sleep. An increase of serotonin levels also impacts your memory, sexual function, mood, appetite, and social behaviors positively too.

Increases dopamine

When you exercise, this helps increase your brain's dopamine levels in order to decrease stress, depression, and other issues. The chemical makes you feel good and it also helps eliminate the feeling of edginess caused by stress.

These are just some examples of how exercise can affect your hormones positively. If you haven't started your own workout routine yet, it's time to start building one. When it comes to hormones and physical exercises, the biggest enemies you have are sitting around and over-exercising. Leading a sedentary lifestyle for too long might throw your hormones off balance. Unfortunately, this has become such an issue these days that scientists have coined the term "Sedentary Death Syndrome" that refers to the detrimental health effects caused by a prolonged sedentary lifestyle.

Over-exercising is just as bad. Doing this increases your stress hormones along with an increased risk of infections, injury, muscle loss, poor recovery, and fatigue. While exercise is recommended, you must give your body enough time in between your workout sessions to reduce stress response and recover properly.

In order to maximize the health benefits of exercise and give your hormone levels a boost, the best combination is cardio workouts and strength training. High-intensity exercises are also ideal, especially when you allow your body to rest for a short while in between. The more intense your workout is, the more hormones your body releases. Another important thing to keep in mind when it comes to exercising is consistency. This helps you maintain a steady flow of healthy hormones in your body.

If it is your first time to exercise, do not rush or push yourself. If your goal is to have a toned body, think of exercise as a journey, not something that would cause changes overnight. The key is to maintain consistency and focus on your health goals. do not make it a "binge," instead, make it part of your lifestyle. For this issue, here are some tips for your hormone fix:

- Be aware of how much time you spend sitting throughout the day—and try to reduce that time. Whenever possible, make the choice to walk more. Simple choices such as this make huge impacts on your health when done consistently.

- Give pilates and yoga a try as these exercise methods offer so many health benefits. These are incredible anti-aging exercises that improve your posture, mood, stress levels, strength, and flexibility. All of these positive health benefits also support the health of your hormones to restore your balance naturally.
- Give high-intensity interval training (HIIT) a try, too. This is especially true if you want to burn fat as it's more efficient compared to aerobic exercises. Apart from strengthening your heart and lungs, HIIT also increases your body's production of human growth hormone that makes you strong and healthy.

Restoring Your Energy Levels

As a team, your hormones work together to keep your body running and provide you with energy. However, your diet, stress, and other factors may cause hormonal imbalances in your body thus, causing your energy levels to drop significantly. When it comes to energy levels, the hormones that are most involved in these are:

Adrenaline

When needed, adrenaline provides your body with instant energy to face the current situation. But when you experience small stressors frequently throughout the day, these may trigger the production and release of adrenaline as well. When this happens, it may leave you feeling depleted instead of energized. To combat this, you may want to try performing activities that relax you for at least 10 minutes a day. Over time, this may reduce the adrenaline spikes your body experiences which, in turn, stabilizes your energy levels.

Cortisol

Although most people know this as the stress hormone, it also helps regulate alertness. This is another hormone that helps give you energy throughout the day. Unfortunately, when you experience stressful situations frequently, this may lead to excessive cortisol levels. When this happens, you may feel tired and have low energy throughout the day then feel alert, wired, and awake at night. To avoid the overproduction of cortisol in your body, make sure that you have a regular sleep cycle and you learn how to minimize your stress.

Insulin

This hormone transports glucose from the bloodstream into your muscles that utilize it for fuel. However, you need to maintain appropriate levels of insulin in order to have stable energy levels. When you have chronically high levels of insulin, this may lead to a reduction in your insulin sensitivity. For this issue, exercise can help you out. When you exercise regularly, your muscles are able to use glucose from your bloodstream without requiring insulin. This helps stabilize your hormonal levels so you can feel more energized throughout the day.

Thyroid Hormones

The thyroid hormones regulate metabolism or how the body produces, stores, and utilizes energy. But when your thyroid hormones are out of balance, this may cause you to feel fatigued. In particular, using plastic containers for your food that contain phthalates and bisphenols tends to throw your thyroid functions off. To combat this, try to stay away from plastic containers and products whenever possible. Instead, opt for those made of paper, metal or glass. If you really have to use plastic containers, do not heat your food inside them as this causes the harmful chemicals to seep into your food.

If you want to enjoy stable energy levels throughout the day, maintaining the balance of these hormones is crucial. For this issue, here are more tips for your hormone fix:

- Take some time each day to unwind—this helps promote healthier hormone function.
- Take care of your gut by consuming foods high in fiber and probiotics.
- Load up on healthy fats as these promote the production of energy-boosting hormones.
- Avoid foods that have inflammatory or reactive effects as these may weaken your endocrine system.
- Limit or avoid starchy and sweet foods as these tend to destabilize your hormone levels. Also, if you're feeling low on energy, try to cut back on high-sugar fruits, legumes, and grains for a period of two weeks. This gives your body the time to restore hormonal balance.
- As much as possible, try to avoid taking medications, both prescription and OTC medications. Opt for natural remedies whenever possible since medications can also cause hormonal imbalances.

Nurturing Your Fertility

For Women

Women need hormonal balance for their fertility. This balance ensures that they get pregnant, they are able to carry their babies to term, and they give birth to a healthy baby without complications. As with all the other functions in the body, there are specific hormones that have an effect on fertility. For women, these are:

Cortisol

The main functions of this hormone in terms of fertility are to increase the levels of blood sugar, suppress the immune system, and aid in the metabolism of protein, fats, and carbohydrates.

DHEA

This is a precursor hormone to estrogen and testosterone. It is crucial for protein repair and building.

Estradiol or E2 estrogen

This hormone is essential for the healthy formation of bones, for gene expression, for the maintenance of healthy levels of cholesterol, and for the formation of the secondary sexual characteristics. It is also crucial for the health of a woman's menstrual cycle.

FSH

This hormone is responsible for regulating the growth, development, and maturation of the body. It also plays an important role in the regulation of reproductive processes.

Luteinizing Hormone

This hormone triggers ovulation along with the development of corpus luteum. It also stimulates cells for them to start producing testosterone.

Progesterone

This hormone is important for healthy bone formation, blood clotting, and libido. It helps with the regulation of the menstrual cycle too while balancing the effects of estrogen. Women require enough amounts of this hormone for their fallopian tubes to function normally. It is also crucial for fertilization and for women to maintain their pregnancies. Another important function of progesterone is that it supports the embryo that develops in the womb of women.

Testosterone

This hormone is found in minimal amounts in women and it supports the building of bones along with a healthy libido.

For Men

Of course, fertility is also important for men. Although women are the ones who get pregnant, there is no chance of this happening when men have issues with their fertility. In men, the hormones involved in fertility are:

- **Cortisol** increase the levels of blood sugar, suppress the immune system, and aid in the metabolism of protein, fats, and carbohydrates.
- **DHEA** helps maintain the levels of testosterone for a healthy sex drive and so men can sustain their erections.
- **Estrogen** is important for sexual arousal and proper production of seminal fluid and sperm.
- **FSH** is responsible for stimulating the primary spermatocytes causing them to divide and form secondary spermatocytes. This hormone plays a crucial role in the initiation of sperm creation.
- **Luteinizing hormone** plays an important role in sperm creation.
- **Progesterone** is important for regulating inflammation responses and the immune system. It also helps improve vascular tone along with other crucial functions.
- **Testosterone** is important for the development of the prostate, testis, and secondary sexual characteristics. This hormone also plays a significant role in reproductive function, erection, libido, and sexual arousal.

For Both Genders

Fertility is important for both men and women. If you feel like you have issues with your fertility, this may be caused by hormonal imbalances. Here are some tips for your hormone fix:

- Learn how to manage your stress more effectively in order to maintain adequate cortisol levels. If you feel particularly stressed, try taking relaxing baths, massages or trying yoga poses that promote fertility.
- Practice meditation and mindfulness as they help promote overall hormonal balance.
- Apart from getting enough sleep, make sure that your sleep is always continuous and restful.
- Quit smoking, drinking excessive amounts of alcoholic and caffeinated beverages, and other unhealthy habits.
- Include adaptogenic herbs in your diet to boost your fertility. Some examples of these herbs that promote fertility are ashwagandha, maca root, chaste tree, and turmeric.

Conclusion: Healthy Hormones for
a Healthy Life!

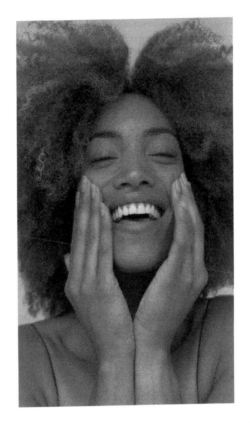

\With everything you have learned about hormones thus far, you may have a more enlightened perspective of these incredible chemical messengers in your body. Whenever you hear the term "hormone," you do not only have to think about women or teenagers having emotional outbursts. Hormones are so much more than that, and you know it.

Hormones control a number of bodily functions; that's why it's extremely important to keep everything in balance. When you experience any kind of hormonal imbalance, it causes a cascade of negative effects on your well-being. Thus, you should always focus on maintaining a steady flow of hormones throughout your system.

In relation to the latter, here are a few more tips to keep in mind:

- Breathe deeply as your cells love oxygen. Breathing deeply also helps reduce the levels of stress hormones in your body.

- Remember that all types of exercise can lower your levels of stress. Find the best type of exercise and stick with it!
- Drink a lot of water as this would keep everything flowing smoothly throughout your body, even your hormones.
- Only eat when you feel hungry and avoid overeating. Listen to your body so your hormones that control digestion won't lose their effectiveness.
- Make sure that you get enough sleep each night and that your sleep is restful and rejuvenating. This will help revitalize your entire endocrine system to keep it functioning at its best.

Our bodies have so many types of hormones, all of which are performing specific functions. Still, scientists are discovering more things about these microscopic wonders. The more they know, the more they will be able to share how we can keep our hormones happy, healthy, protected, and balanced.

Throughout this book, you have learned a lot of information about hormones. Since hormones play an important role in our lives, ensuring their health means that you are ensuring a healthy and happy life too! That's what hormone fix is all about!